PENGUIN BOOKS

Just One More Question

Niall Tubridy was awarded his medical degree from the Royal College of Surgeons in Ireland in 1991. He went on to work in hospitals in Dublin, London, Paris and Melbourne. Since 2004, he has been a consultant neurologist at St Vincent's University Hospital, Dublin. He is also a professor of clinical medicine at University College Dublin.

JUST ONE MORE QUESTION

Stories from a Life in Neurology

NIALL TUBRIDY

PENGUIN BOOKS

PENGUIN BOOKS

UK | USA | Canada | Ireland | Australia
India | New Zealand | South Africa

Penguin Books is part of the Penguin Random House group of companies
whose addresses can be found at global.penguinrandomhouse.com.

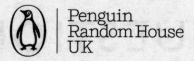

Penguin
Random House
UK

First published by Penguin Ireland 2019
Published in Penguin Books 2020
001

Printed and bound in Great Britain by Clays Ltd, Elcograf S.p.A.

A CIP catalogue record for this book is available from the British Library

ISBN: 978-0-241-98538-0

www.greenpenguin.co.uk

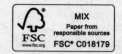

MIX
Paper from
responsible sources
FSC® C018179

Penguin Random House is committed to a
sustainable future for our business, our readers
and our planet. This book is made from Forest
Stewardship Council® certified paper.

To

The Wednesday Barrel Club

When you're reading this account of my life in neurology, you should be aware that while everything told here is true, the raw material has been reconfigured. My experiences of dealings with patients and colleagues have been broken down and reconstructed. Cases are merged, so many of those outlined are composites of different stories, and I have been careful to either omit or change identifying details about patients. If you have been a patient of mine and think you recognize yourself, it is not possible that you could be the patient described in the pages that follow; please be assured that any similarity is coincidental.

'The chief function of the body is to carry the brain around.'

Thomas A. Edison

CONTENTS

1. Early Lessons   1
2. Amnesia by the Seaside   9
3. The Stud   17
4. Santa Visits Barons Court   23
5. First Impressions   29
6. The Big Picture   37
7. Locating the Damage   49
8. Sliding Doors   57
9. All in the Mind?   63
10. Signing Up for Medicine at Seventeen   71
11. The Many Faces of Multiple Sclerosis   79
12. Living with a Label   89
13. A Pain in the Head   99
14. Coppers on a Wednesday Night   107
15. Like Father, Like Son   117
16. Heal Thyself   123
17. The Choker   129
18. Kevin and Aristotle   135
19. The Aftermath   143
20. More than Just a Hiccup   151
21. Burnout   157
22. Off-Balance   163
23. A Hidden Side of Cancer   171
24. Anthony's Story   179

CONTENTS

25. A Day in the Life   191

26. Passing the Baton   201

27. The Price of Saying 'Yes' to the Dress   211

28. Dr Google   217

29. Himself   227

30. A Shaking Palsy   233

31. Tales of the Unexpected   245

32. Doctoring in the Twenty-first Century   259

33. 'Am I Losing It?'   265

34. 'Where Do All the Old People Go?'   275

Conclusion   285

Acknowledgements   291

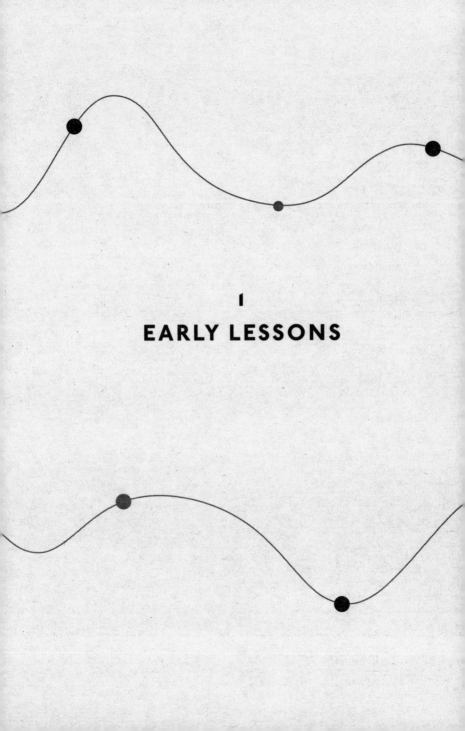

1

EARLY LESSONS

You never forget the first time you tell someone their life is going to change for ever. I was twenty-eight and my patient was just three years younger. While out jogging Jenny had lost the power in her left leg and had gone to see her GP. He sent her to Casualty locally and they sent her immediately to the neurology department at the large London hospital where I was then training. My boss, the consultant neurologist, had been called away, so I had to see her on my own. A nurse helped her into the examining room. By now both of her legs were so weak that even with support she walked very unsteadily.

I was as nervous as Jenny was fearful. I took her medical history and she mentioned that an uncle had multiple sclerosis. This was a red flag because given her symptoms and profile – young, white and female – MS was a very strong possibility. She casually mentioned that she had experienced an episode, a few years before, of blurred vision for a few weeks but had ignored it at the time. I did some routine neurological tests. She had very brisk knee reflexes – a bad sign. When I stroked the soles of her feet her big toes sprang upwards – also a bad sign. In adults the big toe should bend downwards when the sole of the foot is stroked but when the nervous system is damaged it returns to its 'baby state' and goes up instead. So when Jenny's big toes jumped upwards I knew that she had suffered serious nerve damage.

A few weeks later, I had the results of her MRI scan and her brain showed all the markers we expect to see in someone with MS. Though I was confirming to Jenny what we had both strongly suspected, this was still a shattering moment.

'My uncle has been in a wheelchair for as long as I can remember,' she said when I told her. She began to cry.

I said that not all people with MS become wheelchair-dependent. She asked if I could guarantee that she would not and I had to say no.

This was in pre-Google days so patients' knowledge about neurological conditions tended to be anecdotal. That meant, inevitably, that high-visibility worst cases were the ones people knew about. Jenny, naturally, thought of her uncle. She was unaware of all of those with MS who got on with quite normal lives and were not debilitated. It wasn't for Jenny to know that she had a good chance of a better life than her uncle and, hopeful as I was, I couldn't make any promises. All I could hope to do was help her understand her condition, explain the, at that stage rather limited, treatment options available and encourage her as much as possible.

I took a particular interest in Jenny's situation because it was a personal milestone for me – doctors are morbidly excited by their first major diagnosis, and I was no different. Grim though it sounds, young medics' passion for their discipline is what drives their initial efforts to help their patients. Like all jobs, you're pleased to be putting your hard years of study into practice in the real world. You want to tell your friends about your big diagnosis and track the impact of your attempts to help people. Now I felt like a neurologist.

It had taken me a few years to figure out what kind of doctor I wanted to be. Dissecting a brain in the anatomy lab was, well, gruesome. So I knew that surgery was not for me pretty much straight away. I liked cardiology as well, and I was also giving some thought to being a geriatrician. Then in fourth year we were assigned to the hospital wards. This was daunting. Like generations of students before and since, we wandered forlornly around the wards trying to keep out of everyone's way. During ward rounds we would hang around in the background while the real doctors spoke to and examined patients. We loved those teachers who gave us the time to explain things, and those who were the most demanding would always turn out to be the most enthusiastic, and certainly the ones we remembered.

One of my earliest rotations was with the neurology team. Leading the team were two well-known consultants. They seemed to stand head and shoulders above the other physicians – at least in my young eyes. Their clinical acumen was terrific and, with an almost insouciant arrogance, they would appear to take only a few minutes to diagnose a patient. They could always make a complicated diagnosis look easy. There was a significant amount of ego involved, for sure, but underneath the bravado there was great clarity in what they were doing and how they went about it.

So I loved neurology from the start. I loved the logical nature of the history taking and examination. I was amazed by the finely tuned way that neurologists listened to every cadence of a patient's voice; how they watched, all but forensically, every flicker of movement. They were like expert electricians who could find the precise area where the wiring or the bulbs were faulty. And I loved the discussions they would have about unusual cases and how they would argue over one clinical sign after another. Watching from the back of the group of nurses and junior doctors was exhilarating.

Beyond that, I was humbled to learn so much from the patients who were frequently getting a life-changing diagnosis – how they responded emotionally to what life had thrown at them, and how their loved ones watched on in their moments of agony and ecstasy. I thought that nothing could top looking after people whose brains were sick. I saw it as a wonderful way to get to know patients as individuals at what I felt was a deeper level.

Given the appeal of neurology at an existential level, it's curious that I never had any interest in taking up my father's speciality, psychiatry, even though it is undeniable that the two subjects are linked (and now more than ever). I guess I wanted to plough my own furrow. I argued sometimes with my dad about how little, apparently, psychiatrists could do for their patients. Yet that was, and is, a criticism habitually levelled at neurologists.

In those days, and perhaps even still, neurology was seen as a somewhat odd choice. Neurologists have long been considered the intellectual end of medicine – dickie-bow-wearing nerds who seek the esoteric in the simple – but just because you study the brain does not mean you are 'brainy'. I think the reputation of neurologists stems from our student days. With so few drug therapies available when I was training in the early 1990s, it seemed it was all about making a diagnosis and not being able to do very much to actually help people. No wonder it attracted so few of my friends who, understandably, saw this as the point of becoming a doctor.

Jenny was admitted to the hospital so we could assess the best treatment options for her and I would call in to see her twice a day. Along with the tears there was laughter too – there's often laughter in the hospital, and it helps to sustain both doctor and patient through the darker moments of treatment.

Jenny did not appear to have many visitors, which was strange for a young woman from a big family. I asked her about this and she went quiet. She was embarrassed, she told me. She had asked her family not to visit, and told them that the hospital was prohibiting visitors in the first week of her illness. She didn't want them to see her as she was; she knew that they'd look at her and think straight away of the uncle whose life had been changed by the same condition.

Eventually, she told me tearfully that she was getting married in six months' time. 'That's great news,' I said. 'Congratulations!' But it was obvious to us both that her life had changed irrevocably.

I offered to tell her fiancé when he came up to visit. I could see her panic rising as her face flushed with anger. She practically shouted at me, 'Don't you dare!'

'But you have to tell him!' I blurted out in surprise. 'You can't marry someone without telling them the truth?'

How naïve I was.

'He'll never marry me if he thinks I could end up in a wheelchair! Would you marry someone in this position?'

Nearly twenty-five years later I can still see her tear-flecked face and the fury in her eyes. I was young, but not that young. I was in a relationship myself and immediately wondered how I would feel if my girlfriend hid something like that from me. I was almost as furious as Jenny at the thought. This was deceit of the cruellest kind, I felt at the time. But I was young and healthy; here was this young woman at the edge, with the prospect of a lifetime of disability ahead of her, and just to top it off, this heartless doctor was going to reveal her secret to her fiancé. No wonder she was raging, not just with me, but with the world.

I duly promised not to say anything, but I walked away seething. I am still not entirely clear what I was angry at. The lie, or a shaken trust in relationships? How would I *actually* feel if this were my bride-to-be? And then, how would I feel if it were me unable to move my legs, having just been told I had MS? What would I do?

'*Love is not love which alters when it alteration finds,*' quoted the senior nurse when I stormed into the office, mouthing off about Jenny's imminent betrayal.

I was taken aback by her response. She had been a neurology nurse for more years than I had been alive, and had seen the full gamut of emotions that comes with the speciality. She was calm and reassuring with even the most hysterical patient or relative (or junior doctor), and I had a lot to learn from her.

'It is not your job as a doctor to judge people. Whatever the rights or wrongs of her decision, they are her rights and wrongs to make, and not ours.'

'But is it not unfair of her not to tell her fiancé? Is it not my responsibility to explain it to him too?'

'It may seem unfair, but that's nothing to do with us,' she said firmly.

She was dead right, of course: it is not a doctor's responsibility – nor is it even permissible – to share a patient's medical information with anyone else without their say-so. At times this causes consternation, for example when a concerned parent or a spouse calls to discuss things without the patient's knowledge, but it is one of the golden rules of medicine that protects the privacy and confidentiality of the doctor–patient relationship.

It was an early lesson: I had to learn to detach myself from the patient's life and emotional involvement in their care if I was ever going to be able to handle my job of making them better and supporting them in the longer term – which was plenty to be getting on with. I didn't want to become cold and uncaring, but there was a line I would have to learn to tread in the years to come. Most of the time, I would hope to get the balance right, and would just go on to the next problem. But when the sleepless nights start racking up as you ruminate in the small hours about what might become of a patient and their future you realize that you are in danger of crossing the line again.

When I did the ward round with the consultant the next day, I could barely hold Jenny's gaze. I asked the consultant what he thought about her attitude.

'Don't be ridiculous,' he said. 'That's none of our business, and the sooner you realize that, the better.' Then he softened and said that he had 'been there and done that' as a younger doctor, and had come to understand that this was not the right approach to thinking about the patients.

It took a few weeks for me to understand Jenny's decision not to tell her fiancé. I met the young man only once and said hello, but he never asked me any questions and generously thanked me for helping to make Jenny better. They did get married later that year and I met them in the outpatient clinic a year after that. She was doing well, and had suffered no further attacks of MS. I moved away from the hospital, as is the way with the wandering young doctors, and never found out what the future held for this young couple, or whether her MS had ever returned. I am forever grateful for what they taught me and, as a result, how I taught the lesson to generations of young doctors since. It is extraordinary how influential a single patient can be without their ever realizing it. Likewise that wise and patient nurse – I still cherish the moment that we sat down together for a cup of coffee so she could talk some sense into me.

2

AMNESIA BY
THE SEASIDE

'I had breakfast, drove to Dun Laoghaire and went for a walk. I remember nothing of the next six hours.'

'Every time I have an orgasm my head explodes.'

'Last night I saw Santa Claus. He was in a helicopter over my head in the bedroom.'

When I heard stories like these I knew why I would love being a neurologist. To meet people who had just gone from the land of the neurologically well to the neurologically unwell is an endless source of fascination. Ordinary people living their ordinary lives like you and I are suddenly faced with the fragility of their own minds.

I regularly hear the younger doctors make their first diagnosis of an unusual neurological syndrome and, while I love their excitement – and recall my own when at their stage – I have to remind them and myself that rare things are just that: rare. It is unfortunately the way of the world in medicine that what is rare is interesting and nowhere does this apply more than in neurology.

Nathan was a Canadian chef, living in Dublin with his wife of twenty-five years, Janet. They had been settled in Ireland for many years and ran a small restaurant together. It was a good life and he had few cares in the world. He was a creature of habit. His daily routine was to have breakfast with Janet, then a quick shower before setting off for a walk. He would drive to the car park at St Michael's Hospital in Dun Laoghaire, leave the car there and walk the mile or so to the East Pier of Dun Laoghaire Harbour and then walk the pier. On his daily constitutional Nathan liked to reflect on the events of the previous day and plan the menus for the evening ahead.

On this cold February morning, Nathan followed his usual routine and nothing seemed amiss until he got home.

'What time is it?' he asked Janet.

'Oh, about half past ten,' she replied.

After a minute, he asked again. 'What time is it?'

'It's about half ten,' she replied again, assuming he had not heard her the first time.

'But what time is it now?'

Janet turned to face him, exasperated, as he sat at their kitchen table staring into space. Here was yet another moment in their long marriage when he was not listening.

'Are you getting deafer or just ignoring me?' she asked.

She looked closely at his expressionless face for a moment until he spoke.

'What time is it?'

There was no inflection in the question.

'What time is it?' he said again.

'What is wrong with you?' She had been amused and then irritated, thinking that he might be making fun of her. Now she was growing wary.

'What time is it?'

She changed tack, as he seemed to be both speaking and looking into the distance.

'Okay, enough now', she said, raising her voice. 'We have things to do before the restaurant opens.'

'But what time is it?' he said, as if she was not even in the same room. Janet tried to remain calm as she sat down beside him and held his hand.

'Nath, are you okay?'

A dropped beat, a blink of an eye. 'What time is it?'

Her panic growing, she led him to the sitting room. He appeared to be moving normally and his facial expression, though flat, was not asymmetrical and did not appear drooped (she had learned from the radio that this was something to look for if you thought someone was having a stroke). She sat down beside him on the couch.

'Nath, it is me, Janet. Don't you recognize me?'

He looked directly into the eyes of the love of his life. Briefly, she felt she saw him recognize her familiar features.

'What time is it?'

By the time I saw Nathan in Casualty it was three hours since he had had his scrambled eggs and toast with his wife that morning. He looked very calm – almost serene – but his poor wife was in a terrible state. She was trying to hide her sense of fear and panic but could not stop the tears rolling down her face. She held his hand gently and led him through the crowded department as if she was guiding a child around a shopping mall. Her distress did not seem to register with Nathan. He seemed completely oblivious to what was happening.

By now, he had added a second question to the repertoire: 'Where am I?' Having said hello, he asked me, 'Where am I?' I told him he was in St Vincent's Hospital Casualty. This was less than twenty minutes from his home and in an area he knew very well. He looked at me with the same lack of interest in his surroundings.

'Where am I?'

He asked the same question over and over again, only occasionally looping back to 'What time is it?'

It was close to two o'clock that same afternoon when the fog began to lift. The questions continued but the range expanded.

'Where's my car?'

'Where am I?'

'Where's my wife?'

'What time is it?'

Nathan's neurological examination was normal – apart, obviously, from his ability to take in any new information. He could see. He could hear. He could drink the cup of coffee given to him. He could speak. The tone, power and coordination of his limbs were as they should be. His reflexes were all present and his big toes turned downwards when I scratched the soles of his feet. Yet he could not process his circumstances. He was not unlike a small child briefly separated from a parent in a supermarket – perhaps a little less upset but still vulnerable and fearful about possibilities not hitherto imagined.

About an hour later, Nathan suddenly piped up: 'What the hell is going on?' He sounded totally different. Gone was the robotic repetition. The blank-faced automaton was replaced by a playful, smiling, Santa Claus-like figure who reached out his hand to comfort his anxious-looking wife.

'I'm fine, Janet,' he laughed. 'Why all the fuss and what on earth am I doing in St Vincent's?'

Nathan's last memory was asking his wife whether she had wanted some scrambled eggs at the breakfast table that morning. He had no recollection of his shower, the drive to Dun Laoghaire, the walk on the pier in the cold rain, or the drive home. The period of memory loss was about four hours, although he had occasional glimpses of images from the morning. As the day wore on, he recalled getting into the shower and some of the events in Casualty a few hours later.

Nathan's scans and blood tests were all fine. His recovery appeared complete but he would never regain the lost time despite his best attempts.

I have seen hundreds of similar cases over the years, and the existential angst on the faces of people who have had an episode of transient global amnesia (TGA) is always striking. The same is true for the terror on the faces of their loved ones. Their horror is more than justified: a person is cruising through life with nothing but their ordinary hopes and fears when, out of the blue, the bright and funny person they love appears like a child on a long car journey, asking, 'Are we there yet?' again and again.

I can't imagine what went through Janet's mind during that terrifying time. Did she reflect on their courtship, their marriage and their lovely life together? Did she worry about their family business and what was going to happen? Did she look at a future without her best friend? Did she fear that he would be incapacitated and she would have to look after him for the rest of their time together? Possibly all of these things.

The exact cause of such bouts of temporary amnesia remains unknown. After meeting Nathan, my senior colleague mentioned a research paper from the 1970s by his own predecessor at St Vincent's. Dr Martin called the paper 'Amnesia by the seaside', although the phenomenon had been described elsewhere some years previously. It has variously been thought to be due to either a stroke, a seizure or a migraine, but definitive proof of what causes it remains elusive. The unfortunate individual loses their short-term memory and the ability to lay down new memories for up to twenty-four hours. It can be provoked by immersion in water (hot or cold) or extremes of exertion and excitement. This suggests a Valsalva-type manoeuvre (that's exhaling while keeping the mouth closed and pinching your nose or extreme straining to keep the air in the lungs – something you might see weight-lifters do prior to a lift; they do it to keep the lungs inflated and provide greater stability in their torsos), with subsequent congestion of the veins draining the memory centres in the brain, might be the cause. Sometimes MRI brain scans can show a lack of blood flow in the memory centres of the brain but this is variable in my experience. The precise cause remains mysterious.

Transient global amnesia usually occurs in people in their fifties or sixties but can occur in younger folk. Repetitive questions, in an apparent bid to orientate themselves, are often a significant feature. In most other respects the affected person appears to behave normally. It starts abruptly but recovery tends to be gradual. Understandably, those who observe the phenomenon in loved ones suspect they are having a stroke or a seizure.

Cathy went to the All-Ireland Football Final in Croke Park. Having driven up with her parents from Kerry, the excitement for the 26-year-old was enormous. It was only ten minutes into the game when the Kerry fans rose as one to acclaim a spectacular point, and Cathy suddenly forgot everything. She did not know who she was. She did not have a clue where she was or why she was among thousands of strangers looking down on a distant field.

Unsurprisingly, her parents were caught up in the excitement, and it was only at half-time that her father had reason to suspect that all was not well. 'What do you think of the match, Cathy?' he asked.

'Where am I?' she replied distantly. The answer soon afterwards was 'on a hospital trolley'. Cathy's last memory of what was, to that point, one of the most exciting days of her life, was hopping into the shower at home in Listowel before her trip to the All-Ireland.

One Saturday morning Gerald was awoken by his three-year-old grandson. Gerald brought him downstairs to his father in the kitchen and returned to bed to find his wife in an amorous mood. After they had what he later described, blushing, as 'a bit of sex', he could recall nothing of the subsequent three hours of his life.

His wife emerged from a post-coital shower to find her husband grappling with the concept of socks and what on earth he was to do with them. 'What are these?' he asked her, holding them up. He repeated the question dozens of times as she tried to help him dress.

Whether or not he had just had the best sex of his life, Gerald will unfortunately never know. When the couple eventually began to piece together the remnants of his 'trip away from life' later that evening, he kept asking her what it had been like. His wife assured him – albeit in a rather non-committal fashion – that it was up to their usual standards.

I have rarely seen TGA recur, but it can do so. A single isolated episode is the norm and investigations rarely yield any significant abnormalities. What is fascinating is meeting people after such an episode. They marvel at the fine line between health and illness, and how blithe we tend to be about being on the right side of it (as do I, even still, when I witness an episode). Many become anxious that a TGA experience might be a portent of future dementia but this is not the case. Previously confident people can become anxious and less gregarious. While most people manage to bury their worst fears, at least ostensibly, some are never quite the same person again.

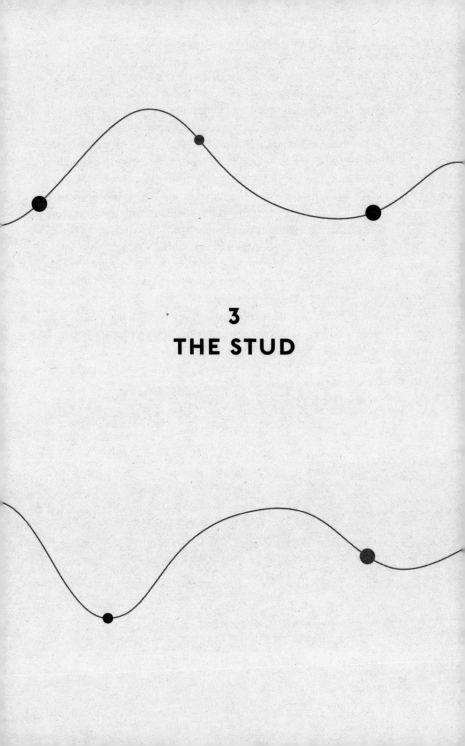

3
THE STUD

'Every time we have sex I get a headache,' Masud murmured sheepishly. 'Not just any headache either, but it feels like I have been hit over the back of the head with a hammer whenever I climax.'

'Every time?' I asked.

I wondered to myself, was this guy making fun of me, or was this potentially leading up to a brain haemorrhage the next time he had sex? With his girlfriend, Sarah, beside him he was self-conscious, of course, but she cajoled him to divulge more. They were both in their mid-twenties and had met only a few months before in a nightclub in London. The attraction was instantaneous, mutual, and extremely lustful. Days at work were missed. They ate only to refuel before the next bout of love-making.

All could not have been rosier until, en route to his third orgasm that day, our young hero developed a searing pain in his neck that rapidly spread throughout his skull. Apologizing for ruining the moment, he held his head in his hands as she tried to comfort him. He walked to the bathroom of her flat, took two paracetamol and lay down. Gradually, and to his immense relief, the pain began to subside.

Within an hour, his urges overcame any fear of the pain he had endured and the coupling began again. This time all seemed well until he actually climaxed (or, as he put it later, 'the money shot was in play, Doctor'). This time the head pain was instantaneous and even more intense than earlier. He said he felt like he had been hit by a brick on the back of his head the moment he reached orgasm. He collapsed on top of his unsuspecting and somewhat distracted partner.

She screamed in fear, but he was able to talk and move his arms, and he could see normally, so he felt he had done the sexual equivalent of pulling a hamstring and told her to relax. The rest of the day's activities were, nonetheless, postponed. He lay down and the intense, sharp pain ebbed to a less severe throbbing one over the next hour or so. Three hours later he was back to himself, if a little more anxious, though he was too proud (or too scared) to share his worries with his girlfriend.

It was with ill-concealed temerity the following morning that Masud decided he would try again. Although apprehensive, given the events of the previous day, Sarah agreed to take things slowly, as the previous few weeks had been the best fun she had had since moving to London the previous spring.

Masud managed to forget his worries altogether for a while. As orgasm approached, he felt a tingle at the back of his head. He ploughed on, only to be felled once again.

Finally, fear won out over embarrassment and he ended up in front of me, a then junior neurologist, a week or two later. 'Every time we have sex I get a headache,' he explained. We were of a similar age but I was in an ill-fitting white coat with a rarely used stethoscope around my neck.

'My dear Dr Tubridy,' the eminent London neurologist who was supervising my training laughed when I presented Masud's story. 'You should try not to get so excited about neurology cases, however interesting they may appear to you to be.' I cannot deny that I had this tendency.

He smiled and explained that what Masud was describing was a classic case of coital cephalgia – otherwise known, predictably enough, as 'sex headache'. He instructed me to request brain scans, and to scan the blood vessels of the brain with an angiogram, to exclude the very rare instances of such headaches having a serious underlying cause such as a cerebral aneurysm.

A week later I went to the clinic waiting room in a very excited state, ignoring my boss's admonitions, to tell Masud and Sarah the good news. The scans I had rushed through as emergencies were all clear, and their lusty endeavours could safely recommence.

To my horror, Masud had not turned up. Had I been wrong? Had the scans missed something disastrous? He still hadn't arrived by the time I'd finished the morning's clinic. My elation at the thought of delivering such good news had swung from fear to anger – anger that I had pulled in favours to expedite these scans (even if I had done it as much to satisfy my own curiosity as for Masud's peace of mind).

I grew more agitated at the thought that he had simply not bothered coming back. How could they not turn up after all I had done for them? How could they deny me my moment of neurological glory? (Now I cringe at the vanity of it!) I decided to phone him.

A groggy Masud answered, doubtless having got over any reservations about further fun, and ignoring my ominous warnings to defer all orgasms until the test results were in.

'Masud!' I could barely contain my anger, 'Where the hell are you?'

'In bed, where do you think?'

In full pushy junior doctor mode, I demanded he come in to see me at once to discuss the precious scans. He apologized and he and Sarah made their way into central London that afternoon.

He was still soft-spoken and self-conscious when we met on this second occasion, but there was something else. He was no longer afraid, but appeared rather bashful. As I started to remind them, self-importantly, of all the trouble I had gone to, Sarah nudged Masud with her elbow.

'Just tell him,' she whispered.

He looked away but obviously something had shifted.

'What is it? What are you not telling me?' I asked, rather too frantically. 'I cannot be expected to do the right thing for you if you are not telling me the whole story. Am I missing something?'

'Go on, you have to tell him,' Sarah pushed. I think she felt sorry now for his slightly psychotic young Irish doctor.

Slowly Masud reached into the pocket of his fleece jacket and produced a small tube shaped not unlike those used for sinus decongestion. He placed it on the desk and I examined it. 'The Stud' was emblazoned on the vial's side. It was a nitrate spray he had picked up in Soho and had surreptitiously administered to the relevant area whenever he was about to perform his next round of sexual gymnastics. As anyone who has taken sprays for angina (cardiac chest pain) knows, these nitrate sprays dilate blood vessels not necessarily confined to the heart and headaches are a common side effect. Poor Masud's performance anxiety had led to him purchasing a safety net of nitrate spray, only to induce severe headaches and maximum pain at what should have been moments of maximum pleasure.

Coital cephalgia is far more common than you might think. Through a combination of embarrassment and fear it is frequently ignored by those afflicted by it, until it becomes truly frightening. I have heard both young and old complain of pain so severe that they fear imminent death.

There are two main types of coital cephalgia. The first occurs before orgasm and tends to mimic a severe tension headache or may even feel like a migraine (indeed, many people with either type of sexual headache have a history of migraine). It comes on gradually over a matter of minutes and may relate to muscle spasms in the head and neck. The second occurs almost exactly at the point of orgasm and is described by patients as the worst headache they have ever had. We use a similar phrase when people present with 'thunderclap' headaches that can be an ominous sign of a blood vessel rupturing and bleeding in the brain (called a subarachnoid haemorrhage). This is a life-threatening type of stroke due to bleeding into the spaces surrounding the brain. When presenting initially, sex headaches are investigated as a possible brain haemorrhage until proven otherwise.

Only a third of patients will survive a subarachnoid haemorrhage with good recovery, another third will survive with neurological disability and one third will die. In some studies, as many as 10 per cent of people presenting with a subarachnoid haemorrhage report sexual intercourse as a precipitating event. So while it's easy to snigger at Masud's story, neurologists take sexual headaches very seriously indeed. As for those who routinely respond to a sexual overture with 'Not now, I have a headache' – that might be a job for a different type of doctor.

4
SANTA VISITS BARONS COURT

Harold thought it odd the first time he stared out of his kitchen window in Barons Court in London and observed two young boys playing together in his small back garden. He did not recall having seen them before and didn't think that his elderly neighbours on either side had grandchildren. That these two urchins – for that is what they looked like to Harold – were wearing clothes that would not have been out of place in a Victorian novel was even more unusual, he would think only later that evening. A most cordial and benign man of seventy-three years, Harold concluded that these young boys were not causing any trouble and so he would leave them to his garden, and went about his day.

Over the next few weeks he became only faintly unnerved when the two boys returned to his garden more regularly. As time wore on they were now often accompanied by young girls, also dressed in noticeably drab clothes of a different era. When he would try to gain their attention by gently knocking on the kitchen window, the children seemed oblivious to his presence. In fact, it dawned on him that the strange children dressed in grey were playing noiselessly together.

His interest was further piqued when a group of ten or more children gathered in his garden on a dull London morning dressed as medieval knights. They looked like a children's version of an old Monty Python sketch, he laughed to himself. While they were not disturbing him unduly, and had made no mess of his well-kept lawn nor caused any damage to his vegetable patch, he decided to approach them. He unlocked the back door that led to his garden. By the time he had shut the door behind him and turned to face the mini-medieval knights, they had disappeared.

Harold's wife, Edith, had passed away two years previously, and the last three years of their time together had been tough on both of them. Edith's lost keys and misplaced scarf had evolved quickly over a single year into an inability to find her way home from the local Tesco. Harold had tried his best to cover poor Edith's tracks, but eventually he could no longer trust himself to protect her from herself. He had visited her twice a day for the next two years in the local nursing home.

Looking back now on Edith's descent into her own private amnestic world, Harold started to worry that he too was developing the dreaded Alzheimer's. Yet, he reassured himself, he had no other memory problems. The bills were paid on time, he enjoyed (and remembered enjoying) meeting his old friends for bridge on Tuesday evenings, and, although he struggled to actually see some of the cards at times, he was perfectly able to follow or recall the gossipy conversations of the previous few games.

After a few days of spring-like weather, his street urchins and medieval knights had not turned up, so he reasoned he had simply been under the weather or that his new blood-pressure medication had caused these aberrations in his garden.

All was fine for a few weeks and, not one to bother doctors with trivialities, Harold decided to dismiss it from his mind. It was only when he awoke one night at about two o'clock in the morning to see Santa Claus in a helicopter ghosting over the wardrobe in his bedroom that Harold finally decided to seek medical help.

I saw Harold in the outpatient clinic in Charing Cross Hospital. He could not have been more gentle or kind to me. He tolerated my incessant questions with a smile. He was a very healthy 73-year-old retired schoolteacher. He never smoked, and rarely drank alcohol. There was no history of Alzheimer's in his family, and from his eloquent but succinct responses Harold was patently in full control of his cognitive faculties.

Surprisingly, he seemed untroubled by most of the 'visions', as he referred to them. It was the arrival of Santa Claus that had frightened him into attending his GP, who sent him to our neurology clinic.

He cleaned his glasses as we spoke and asked whether I thought he might need a new prescription. He told me he had had cataract surgery a year or so before, and that he also used drops for early glaucoma.

Harold was presenting with a classic example of Charles Bonnet syndrome. This is usually caused by damage to the visual system such as by glaucoma, cataracts or macular degeneration. It can also be due to damage to the brain areas concerned with vision when the wiring connecting the eyes and the visual area of the brain – called the occipital cortex – is disrupted. It is thought that when the visual input to the brain becomes less than clear – literally because you can't see well or when a part of the brain to do with sight is damaged – surrounding areas of brain take over from their ailing neighbour, but they don't always succeed. In other words, parts of the brain begin to 'make up' images to replace the indistinct images it is receiving.

When they were asked directly, up to 15 per cent of people with impaired vision reported this astonishing phenomenon, which tends to occur in older people because their vision is more likely to be impaired, although it is not exclusive to the elderly. People are slow to report these visual hallucinations for fear their friends and relatives will think them mad or take it as a sign that they have started to develop dementia. Like Harold, they soon become accustomed to the bizarre visions, and some people even begin to find them comforting.

Apart from reassuring patients about what is taking place, and that they are not going mad, mostly treatment addresses the cause of the visual impairment – say, cataracts or glaucoma – and anti-epileptic medications can also help.

It is intriguing to listen to people describing hallucinations of any kind. I saw a retired nurse who had developed high blood pressure and kept seeing the cast of *Fawlty Towers* in a mosaic pattern across her living-room wall. Another man described intricate patterns moving in waves across his bedspread. And yet another began to see the world and the people around her in miniature form (micropsia). Sometimes the images are recognizable scenes from a person's past, but more often they make no sense at all to the patient or anyone else. One cannot but wonder if there is not a vault of visual memories buried deep within all of us only to be released when our brains break down.

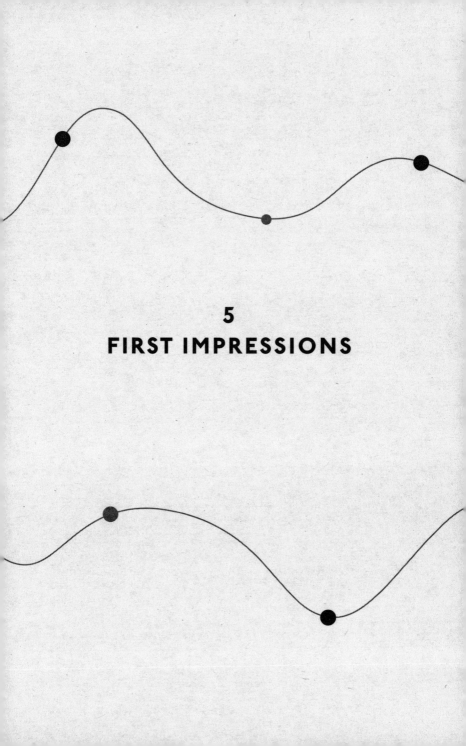

5

FIRST IMPRESSIONS

While rare and colourful cases captivated me as a young doctor, before long I came to understand that the rhythm and shape of my working life would be formed by the commonplace at least as much as, if not more than, the exotic. Of course, in neurology the seemingly commonplace can be devastating. Conditions such as MS and Parkinson's disease change people's lives dramatically; others, like motor neuron disease are usually death sentences. So, while the daily business of being a neurologist might have less excitement than I anticipated, it has greater depth and richness.

Each week I meet at least twenty new patients, and up to 100 others who are attending for regular review. On Tuesday morning the neurology clinic receive more than thirty people for review. Appointments are booked every fifteen minutes with myself or a neurology registrar from 8 a.m. I will usually start before that for the early arrivals. The old 'the doctor will see you now' – the condescending call from a loyal secretary of many years to the next poor patient waiting in the cold and damp waiting room to see the great doctor – is rarely heard any more. No one would put up with such a lofty turn of phrase now, and rightly so. Instead, our receptionist will get the patient's file ready and, if I do not know the patient already, I will look at the GP's referral letter. Once I have the essence of why they've been referred, I will go out to the waiting room and call them in myself, always by their formal title.

I once called a middle-aged man, whom I had never met before. He was barking away into his mobile, upsetting everyone else. He turned nonchalantly towards me when I called his name.

'How are ya, horse?' he shouted over his shoulder as he stomped past me. Here was a confident man, and he wanted everyone to know it.

Most patients nod to their loved ones, who mouth 'good luck', and quietly make their way across the room. I shake hands and introduce myself. From this initial engagement I get a sense of what the appointment is going to be like. Whether it's 'How are ya, horse?' or 'Good morning, Doctor', this moment can be very telling. There are as many kinds of first meeting as there are people in the waiting room. It's a combination of what's going on in patients' heads and their baseline disposition. For some, a weak leg means they will be in a wheelchair and unable to care for their children. For others, they feel they are probably wasting my time fussing over an old rugby injury that has simply raised its head after many years. So, depending on their outlook, some will shake my hand with confidence – or, indeed, squeeze the life out of it to confirm their belief that they're as hale and hearty as ever – while others can barely raise their gaze to meet mine. And, yet, to all appearances, the confident man may be just as fearful as the quiet one, so I try not to make assumptions based on either approach.

There are a few other things that I look out for when I call a patient from the waiting room. Do they faff about to pick up their things and come in (not keen on being here) or rush in (too keen on being here)? Many a follow-up patient in the afternoon clinic will have bags from the posh shops of Dublin, as their annual visit has become a daytrip to the big city; perhaps shopping distracts them from the business at hand. Have they missed previous appointments, and do they apologize for doing so? This may seem terribly judgemental, as I don't know my patients personally, but that's precisely why it's important. Taking note of a patient's little quirks helps to build a picture of their personality, and will help me figure out how best to attempt to relax them as they enter the consulting room. It also helps me to understand how afraid people are. The very concerned come hours before they are due to be seen, like myself going to the airport in fear of missing a flight. Furious gum-chewing might indicate a pre-doctor smoke to calm the nerves. The less concerned arrive, check in and go and get a coffee. The fresh cappuccino placed firmly on the doctor's desk suggests an airy confidence that nothing is wrong as far as they are concerned; the truly worried rarely think of coffee when their long-awaited appointment has finally arrived. Some people are serially late, and nearly always the ones who take up the most time when you are at your lowest ebb at the end of a busy clinic.

How someone dresses when going to see the doctor can be instructive too. Missed bits of unshaved facial hair on a man's chin may suggest a lack of feeling on one side of the face; a tremor might lead to multiple nicks while shaving, some fresh, some healed. A single scuffed shoe might point to a long-standing foot drop and an incompletely buttoned shirt suggests frustration at failing manual dexterity. All are potential indicators of neurological dysfunction – but, of course, they may also be nothing.

The next step is to direct the patient to the consulting room. 'First on the left, please.' I'll hold out my hand to indicate the way, so that they will lead on, the better to see how they walk. Many a diagnosis of Parkinson's is all but made by the time someone reaches the consulting-room door. In most cases an expressionless face on greeting, a shuffling gait and a reduced swing of one arm as they take the few steps towards the consulting room is more than enough information to know what is going on.

Other problems can reveal themselves in that hallway; some stroll right past the open door on the left and start opening doors to the right. True, some are just too nervous to take in an instruction as basic as 'first on the left', but if nerves don't seem to be a problem, I immediately worry about cognitive function and dementia. An alarmed husband or wife will have become used to such mistakes over the preceding weeks or months and will know to guide their spouse to the room. When I see these behaviours, and we have yet to sit down, the possibilities are clear and the tenor of the conversation is set.

The next half an hour can be like a dance. How to tell them what they already most likely suspect? Patients rarely ask straight out, in the hope that they are wrong, so it's a question of gauging their state of mind.

Sometimes it's not the patient's behaviour but who they've come with that helps the doctor. When young Irish women arrive with both parents I guess that MS is the big concern. Fear of MS is deep-rooted in the Irish psyche for reasons I have never been able to fully understand. It seems to be taken as read that any young woman with neurological symptoms has MS until proven otherwise. It's true that multiple sclerosis is very common in Ireland, and that it is more common in women than in men. A lot of people I see will recall an aunt, a distant cousin or a grandmother who had the condition, and the stories of their original symptoms seem to enter into family lore for generations. This probably dates back to when treatments weren't as advanced as they are now and we saw more young people in wheelchairs. Also, decades ago, in a time before MRI scans could provide more precise diagnoses, MS was often given as the most likely explanation for neurological problems of all kinds. But to this day non-medical folk regularly assume any neurological disability in young people, particularly women, to be MS.

I'm not sure at what age anyone should go to the doctor on their own, but it surprises me how often someone in their thirties (or even older) will be accompanied by their parents – but not their spouse. Is there a problem in the patient's marital relationship that is manifesting as a psychological symptom – such as arm or leg weakness or persistent pins and needles? Or are they so scared that they have something serious – like MS – that they don't want to tell their spouse?

And how much is there to read into a teenager arriving with one parent and not the other? Has there been a separation or divorce that has led to the teenager becoming stressed and presenting with neurological symptoms, or is the other parent just at work? As extreme – or over-analytical – as it may seem, I have to consider these questions, as not infrequently I will see young men and women with neurological symptoms but yet I can find nothing abnormal when I examine them. This is where it is critical to try to explore any other problems they might have in life – in work, at home, in their relationship – as external stress can lead to the development of physical symptoms. It is, of course, as easy to read too much into a situation as it is to miss some of these flags of family dynamics, so it's a careful balancing act based on listening to and observing the patient and their loved ones.

Some patients come alone, which, if they are worried about dementia, most likely means we'll both have an uplifting consultation. After all, if they have scheduled the appointment and made their way on their own, it's pretty unlikely to be dementia, even if they have been losing their keys or forgetting people's names more than usual. In clinics that can be full of sad stories and dire news, reassuring people that it's natural to forget things as they head back home is a relief to doctor and patient alike.

Having got them into the examining room, I invite people to remove their coats and hats and to sit down. Addled patients will fuss over unbuttoning their jacket and where to hang it, or hesitate over which chair (of two) to sit in. I've seen really stressed patients sit in my chair, which lightens the mood when they realize what has happened. The jacket removed, it is often thrust into the hands of the patient's partner. Some partners make a point to say that they are only there as support; the ones who promise that they are under strict instructions to keep quiet are inevitably the most loquacious. They can't help themselves, but I'm generally glad, as stressed patients can find it hard to remember anything, as if they were in the *Mastermind* chair, so a chatty, open partner can help to fill in the blanks.

I always explain what I plan to do: 'I'm going to ask you lots of questions, as doctors do, but the first few are just a checklist of things to make sure I don't miss anything basic.'

I will routinely have a few medical students with me in the clinic, and always ask before we go into the room whether the patient or their family minds the students being there to give them the option of saying they would rather they were not. Most patients do not mind ('we all have to learn' is their understated and generous response) and some enjoy teaching the students. Others like the attention of a group of doctors (as they perceive it) and feel they are getting the benefit of more than one medical opinion.

And some put on a performance for the students. They see it as an opportunity to indirectly criticize either the doctor personally or the health service as a whole. '*They couldn't tell what was going on for years and it was only after a great effort on my part did I get them to listen.*' I just try to side-step the criticism by bringing the focus back to their health today. These uncomfortable moments are a way people have of asserting their authority when they feel they have been hard done by, by doctors in the past. In fairness, it can be the case that they are right and they have had less than good care so it is best just to listen and hope that if they get a chance to let off a bit of steam that will be the end of it, allowing us to get back to the problem at hand.

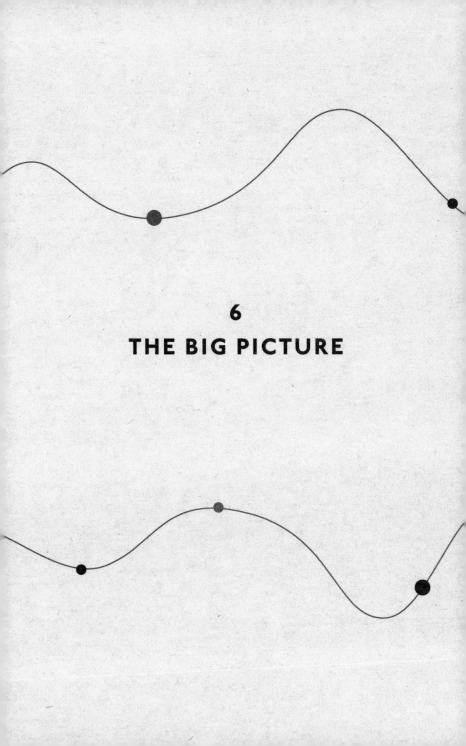

6

THE BIG PICTURE

Shortly after his cancer diagnosis, the journalist Christopher Hitchens wrote of his moment of deportation 'from the country of the well across the stark frontier that marks off the land of malady'. This struck a chord with me and I realized how useful that idea could be when questioning nervous and anxious patients at their first consultation. The sense of being there at the moment that a patient's life changes utterly is a critical starting point in trying to deduce the subsequent diagnosis.

A good narrative is the key to getting and relaying a patient's medical history, as it is with any story. The cadence of the illness is like a musical score. Did the change occur insidiously or abruptly? Has it been progressing or is it a single hit causing static disability? Is it recurring and what factors seem to either provoke it or help alleviate the symptoms?

In meeting patients for the first time, we start with what brought them to see a doctor. It can be something like a numb hand that does not resolve itself, or a weak leg that, after a few miles on a regular walk, refuses to obey their commands to continue as normal. A well-prepared patient will have pondered when that problem began and how it has evolved from the time they originally noticed it. Many will have written down a timeline and be able to tell me who else they have seen about it before coming to me. If they have already had a scan they will bring a copy of it and any other results of tests performed by their GP. If they cannot remember all of the details they might bring someone with them to help clarify the development of their symptoms.

In contrast to all that, I meet some people who tell me they have no idea or can't remember why they have been referred (some waiting times are so long these days this is sadly far more common than you might imagine). The memory plays tricks on us all and we do not recall precisely when we developed any sort of symptom. Yet it still strikes me as a little strange when people have so much difficulty recalling the onset of their neurological symptoms. After all, they had been perfectly well at some point, and then they were not. How can they not remember when they went from one state to the other? Is it a form of denial when we get sick that we say to ourselves 'It's nothing' and plough on, hoping things will just resolve themselves? Or is it so intimidating sitting in front of a doctor that your mind goes blank (as so many patients tell me is the case)? Are they fearful that by revealing all of their symptoms their darkest worries about their illness might be realized?

The moment we consider ourselves sick has particular relevance in the neurology history as initially symptoms may be very subtle. Oftentimes people will have seen a range of specialists before being referred to a neurologist. A weak leg is blamed on a bad back and an orthopaedic opinion is sought (although in Ireland this can be after appointments with a chiropractor, an osteopath, an acupuncturist and even various 'healers' dotted around the country). Others will have had their eyes tested thinking that it is a case of needing new glasses to remedy blurred vision, or their ears examined in the hope that having the wax removed will cure persistent unsteadiness.

In my experience, with enough coaxing, the person will be able to go back to the exact moment they realized something was not right – even if it was many years before. It may be a stumble on a familiar footpath outside the local shop, a missed kick during their Wednesday game of five-a-side or a dropped fork at dinner. It was easy to laugh it off as clumsiness at the time, but many a patient will have been aware deep down, even then, that all was not well. This can go on for months and, in some cases, years. They convince themselves there is nothing wrong in between each stumble or trip. But no matter how hard they try to put it out of their mind, fear will fester in the small hours.

Conversely, others had no reason to think that this minor incident was anything but an isolated event as an extraordinary amount of time can pass before a 'second hit' occurs. It is then that they realize that the incident was not a one-off. Whichever way the person's mind works, eventually something clicks and they decide they cannot ignore the problem any longer.

Taking a good neurological history can appear terribly intrusive and is a very personal thing for patients. It is engrossing to see how vulnerable even the most worldly person can become in front of a doctor – like a child in a confessional, they don't want to say the 'wrong' thing lest the penance they are asked to pay is too great. Reading a patient's body language tells you so much, and listening carefully to their answers to your questions enables you to put together the jigsaw of their lives so you have a context for their medical complaint.

My first question, a simple one, is how old they are. The responses are always instructive, and, funnily enough, people rarely just give a number. Some refer to their next birthday ('fifty-four next April') rather than state their actual age now. It is lovely to hear older folk refer to their age as 'seventy-nine and a half', accompanied by a wink – 'the half is very important at my age!' Answering by birth year – 1946, say – is typical among those who prefer to no longer celebrate birthdays. I'll push: 'Well, if you were born in 1946, how old does that make you now?' I have to judge between nervousness and cognitive decline before pressing any further. Sometimes a patient will look to their spouse for the answer, and so my concerns about dementia will rise.

Another on the list of basic questions is whether the patient is right- or left-handed. We also have to ask if they are right-handed 'originally'. It was a feature of schooling in Ireland and elsewhere not too many years ago that left-handed children (in Irish, you'd have been called a *ciotóg*) were forced to write with their right hands. If, like me, you're right-handed, then there is about a 95 per cent chance that the left side of your brain is dominant. The left hemisphere of the brain controls the right side of the body, and in right-handed people the left brain determines most of our ability to speak. For left-handed people it is about 60/40. That is, 40 per cent of left-handers will be right-brain dominant, and 60 per cent will be left-brain dominant. This is critically important in most brain conditions but is most obvious in stroke. If I have a stroke in my left brain, I am likely to develop right arm and leg weakness and I might well have great difficulty forming sentences or even understanding what is being said. If I have a stroke in my right brain, I will have left-sided weakness, but my speech will generally be well preserved. So it is important to define right- and left-handedness at the onset of every history. If someone is struggling with their speech, then we usually know where to start looking for the fault in the brain with a view to trying to fix it.

Beyond this, I'll go through other health issues. Even if they present with, say, a weak leg, I'll ask about their vision, speech and ability to swallow, and then their bladder and bowel function. I do this not only to make sure I don't miss any symptoms that may be relevant to their weak leg, but also because many patients typically don't volunteer symptoms beyond the leg. They do so either because they think a problem swallowing, for example, is unconnected to the leg and, being considerate, don't want to waste my time with a laundry list of minor ailments, or they're already fearful that the symptoms are all connected, and the problem is far worse than they suspected.

The next question I tend to ask is what, if any, regular medication a person is taking. This will influence any medication I might later consider, to avoid drug interactions, but it will also flag the patient's other illnesses. People may say that they're not on any medications – 'we don't do tablets in our family' is a frequent, proud refrain – and later mention that they regularly take aspirin, or a blood-pressure drug and a cholesterol drug. Sometimes they've been taking them for so long it is second nature and they don't see them as medicine at all. Young women can be the very same when it comes to the contraceptive pill.

The list of medications can vary greatly from one person to the next, and the lists can be lengthy. The latter is the bane of both patients' and doctors' lives. Some people are very organized and come with colour-coded spreadsheets of their tablets past, present and – potentially – future. Others bring worn-out boxes and bottles of assorted tablets. The expectation is that the doctor will know what these little blue and brown pills are, but this is rarely the case, and an inordinate amount of time is spent going through the names of each medication, the dose and the times at which they are taken. How some people remember to take so many combinations of drugs is staggering. I admit to rarely remembering to finish a prescribed course of antibiotics – you should, mind you! – and marvel at patients who can take thirty or more tablets a day at the right time and in the right sequence without making an error. It is, to my mind, a remarkable achievement in itself.

The tablets they take that are not prescribed can be even trickier to unpick. Many people I see with chronic headaches are taking a combination of over-the-counter painkillers every day. 'What do you take when you get a headache?' I might ask. 'Oh, just paracetamol,' they reply. 'The odd time I have to take a Nurofen . . . or a Difene . . . and, if it's really bad, I take a Solpadeine.' Gradually it dawns on the patient that they're taking a painkiller every few hours, every day. This inevitably causes what's known as medication overuse headaches: the treatment has become the disease.

Similarly, most patients don't consider complementary therapies or vitamin tablets to be 'medication', but can be consuming them in vast quantities (though in numerous studies many of these – particularly homeopathic remedies – have been shown to have little or no medical impact at all). However, once again understanding what people are taking (even if it may be entirely inert), and why, can be crucial in getting the bigger picture.

When I have the right list and doses of medication, I can usually discern the general health of a patient. Blood-pressure tablets can cause all sorts of problems like dizzy spells, and anti-angina tablets can cause headaches. Some people start taking aspirin because a friend suggested it would be a good idea; others believe that their cholesterol medication will free them from future heart and stroke problems. When I see a person taking medication for their blood pressure, cholesterol and diabetes, for example, then their neurological problems could all be due to a stroke; if there is a problem in the blood vessels in their heart, then their symptoms may well be due to a similar blood-vessel problem in the head. Frequently it may be the medication causing the symptoms.

Long-term conditions like high blood pressure or diabetes are an important part of a patient's basic medical history, but such illnesses may be so integral to people's lives that they forget to mention them until asked. Diabetes is a common condition both in Ireland and throughout the world, and I am in awe of the people who live with it, particularly those who develop it at an early age. The young teenagers who have to inject themselves regularly with insulin and monitor their own blood sugars several times a day are incredible. Teenage years are notoriously problematic for us all, but it is truly admirable to get through them while managing a chronic condition. Diabetes, like all ongoing conditions, is of interest to neurologists for several reasons. It can affect the peripheral nerves and lead to neuropathic pain in the hands and feet, or persistent pins-and-needles sensations. Diabetes can also affect the eyesight, among other things, so careful monitoring of blood sugars is vitally important.

I also still ask whether someone has ever suffered from tuberculosis (TB), which is still prevalent in some parts of the world. Thanks to Dr Noel Browne and his successors, who helped bring an almost epidemic condition under control in Ireland in the 1950s and 1960s, TB is becoming increasingly irrelevant in the Irish population. I'm sure he would smile to hear younger people ask me, 'What's TB?'

One of the most interesting and, in many instances, informative components of a patient's stories is their social history, but it requires delicacy. As students we were taught to ask whether someone is married, has children, smokes, or drinks alcohol. These days a more nuanced approach is required. I will still ask a patient if they are married; if they say no, I'll ask whether they have a partner or any children. This can be very helpful in working out what social and financial stresses a person is under without having to ask directly, though some guesswork may be needed. A young woman living with two or three children without other support might well be suffering from stress, for example, leading to chronic sleeplessness and headaches. An older man living alone whose children have emigrated may be lonely, looking for reassurance that his mild memory lapses do not signify incipient dementia and the need for a nursing home.

At times asking personal questions produces heart-breaking answers – how to respond when a patient, already concerned for their health, tells me that they had three children and now have two? To ask what happened seems intrusive, not to ask seems uncaring, but tragedy can be a root cause of an apparent medical problem. The death of a child haunts parents and siblings for ever, and it is a wonder to me how they manage to carry on. But carry on they do, and it can be an unpleasant part of my job to heap further distress on these people when giving them a diagnosis of, say Parkinson's, when they think life has already thrown all that it can at them.

Occasionally the conversation takes a direction that provides an awkward insight into people's home lives. How many underlying tensions does attending a doctor lay bare within families, I often wonder. When an Irish husband says he likes a glass of wine with dinner, his wife may laugh: 'More like a bottle!' And so the row begins. How a relationship is going is ceaselessly absorbing during a neurology consultation, and completely relevant. A couple's level of affection or lack thereof quickly becomes palpable as they hold hands or otherwise reach out to each other as I divulge good or bad news or, alternatively, make no contact whatsoever with their loved one. It's all in how people sit beside each other (legs crossed, arms folded, staring ahead), or how one dominates the conversation even though the other one is the patient – the man who will talk over his wife and try to engage in a laddish conversation while relating his own medical insights, or the wife who will report that the husband sitting beside her complaining of a shake was always nervous and never had any get up and go. This can be deeply uncomfortable and I end up pondering what they talk about in the car on the way home.

Some couples have clearly stopped communicating years earlier, and when I ask the Liverpool football fan who has not missed a match on TV for years who the star player of the team is at the moment, he might laugh it off to avoid answering, but when he doesn't know the answer and his wife says, 'But that's what you talk about all the time!' you can then see the implications dawning and panic setting in. Because she switches off at home it's only in this formal setting, talking to a doctor, that she has registered how much ground he has lost.

It never ceases to intrigue me how two people can live together, day in day out, and not notice their other half fading away before their eyes. In many cases it will turn out that an emigrant son or daughter returning at Christmas has been the catalyst for a visit to the GP and hence to a neurologist. When adult children haven't seen a parent in a while they more readily spot changes that have crept up gradually and remained invisible to the other parent. Having been an anxious emigrant for many years myself when my father was ill, I tend to feel for the worriers sitting in the coffee shops and bars of Dublin Airport on 2 January, wondering what will become of their parents (and, perhaps, what will become of themselves when they grow older, so far away from their family).

Work, of course, brings with it a great deal of stress for many, and their sleeping patterns can bear this out. None of us can function adequately with chronic sleep deprivation, and I often see people with headaches and concentration difficulties as a result.

Young lawyers make stimulating case studies in the neurology clinic. They can seem very confident to begin with. They are used to being in control so conceivably feel uncomfortable when the roles are reversed. Many appear to think doctors are somewhat fearful of dealing with lawyers (in truth we may well be). One young man, when I asked what he did, replied, 'I keep you guys out of jail' – that consultation went well. Some will ask to record the conversation we have, which takes the passive out of passive-aggressive. Others will ask to see the notes I have just written while taking their medical history. It seems they are concentrating more on the mechanics of the consultation than the point of it.

There is nothing to hide and I have no problem with people requesting the notes or even recording the conversation. And, yet, I have to admit to feeling that this leads to a level of defensiveness that breaks the unspoken bond of trust you hope you would have when working as a doctor. In the end, anyone can request to review his or her medical notes so it is hardly the third secret of Fatima. The nature and tone of the requests may affect the tenor of the conversations and the mutual sense of trust between doctor and patient. I realize that my lingering reservation is probably a generational thing. It's also verging on irrational as nothing in their files should surprise or upset patients. Like many institutions, in previous times medicine was hierarchical and had a reflexive culture of secrecy. Even when I was training, patients' files were considered to be for medics' eyes only. Sometimes medics would make observations about patients' demeanour or social circumstances – notes they felt would give colleagues insights into a patient's likely progress or challenges they might face in following a course of treatment. Nowadays, of course, such subjective views do not go into files (which is not to say they are not formed: we are only human, after all), so no patient should be startled to read anything in their file.

Not surprisingly, dealing with colleagues can also be tricky, and when neurology is not their chosen speciality there is a thin line between appearing condescending and making too many assumptions about what your colleague does or does not know about the mechanics of the brain.

After asking whether there is a family history of any ailments, I would ask everyone whether they smoke, drink or do drugs. These questions are not to be judgemental: I'm not about to give patients a lecture about the evils of substance use or misuse. I need to know purely because smoking, drinking or drug-use may have pertinent neurological implications.

The drugs question always raises a smile among the older generation, but I have been caught out on a few occasions by a middle-aged, middle-class, golf-club-attending heroin user, so I ask everyone. For smoking, the answer is rarely straightforward.

'I used to smoke but gave it up.'

'Good for you,' I say. 'When did you give them up?'

'Last week,' goes the embarrassed reply.

When a life-long smoker gives up seemingly out of the blue it may be quite telling. Ask enough questions, past the 'Oh, I was sick of them', or 'Cigarettes are getting too expensive', and you'll find a friend or a parent who has died recently from a smoking-related illness. Or a coughing fit one morning that scared the life out of them. Stopping smoking suddenly is one way that frightened patients try to wrest back control of their health. In neurology, the insidious nature of certain conditions can be ignored to the point where people can't recall when they first became aware that something was wrong, but if it coincided with giving up smoking you can be sure that, at least subliminally, they were preparing themselves for something bad, usually cancer.

Anyone who has drunk too much of an evening will appreciate that one's memory the next day can be flawed. Drinking to excess in the longer term can lead to chronic memory problems, to the extent that heavy drinkers may even appear to have early dementia. It's easy to get a bit unsteady on your feet after a few too many drinks, but in the long term the balance centre of the brain (the cerebellum) will start to degenerate, possibly leading to a permanent state of unsteadiness. As a result, how much and how often a person drinks is of some importance in the neurological history.

There are subtler questions, too; I may ask if a person likes to read and, if so, what they're reading at the moment. 'Oh, he reads all the time,' the spouse will say, but the patient with memory problems won't be able to recall the book they're currently reading. (Some lie and say that they like to re-read books, and proceed to regale me with excerpts from *Wuthering Heights*, which they actually last read in school thirty years before.)

It may seem cruel to put already sick patients under the microscope like this but a neurology consultation has to get to the root of a problem. A neurologist needs a panoramic view of a patient's circumstances, not just of the weak or shaky hand. We need the big picture of their daily lives, and any changes they've detected. Of course, doctors can read too much into a given situation, but after the checklist is complete – social history, family history, medication, drug allergies, chronic diseases, previous medical history – we finally get to the actual reason why a person came to see me.

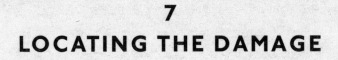

7

LOCATING THE DAMAGE

I love the flow of the neurology exam. Listening to the heart is in and of itself beautiful but limited. Listening to and examining the respiratory system or laying your hands on an abdomen are also interesting but nothing, in my view, compares to the long-playing record that is the well-performed neurology exam. From my student days I found the theatre of it instantly appealing. But quite apart from the flowing aesthetic, the realization of how we move, talk and even think is thought-provoking on an existential level.

A careful observation of each patient's gait is still my favourite part of the process – though it may not be the patient's favourite, particularly if they're walking in front of student doctors. When I was training we would stand like a small army and watch the patient walk the length of the ward corridor and back as if they were on a catwalk.

There then follows an intricate examination of twelve cranial nerves on either side of our head that orchestrate how we see, speak, smell, smile, blink, nod and hear, among other things. This part of the exam also looks at how we eat, how we swallow and even how we move our tongues. It is always mind-boggling to see the intricate ways that these things we take for granted when well can go wrong with the smallest of brain insults. A broken wire here can lead to a dropped face, or an infection there can cause the whole system to collapse.

The examination then moves on to the limbs, examining the motor system connecting our brains to our hands and feet, and then the sensory system running in the opposite direction. I always see it as a railway line that runs from the right brain to the left foot and from the left brain to the right foot. From head to toe the examination looks at the fidelity of the train track. Is it intact and, if it is not, whereabouts has the train been derailed? Was it on the outbound trip or the return journey?

Motor testing assesses the power and tone of each of the muscle groups. It is designed to establish the integrity, or otherwise, of the wiring or neural tracts that run from the brain to our hands and feet. Testing involves a set of simple dance-like moves that, when a patient is showing symptoms of neurological disease, can look a little like a wrestling match. I grasp the patient's arms and legs gently at various points and move the limbs in different directions to assess muscle tone. I then wield a tendon hammer – a long stick with a round rubber head – to elicit the reflexes. You could visualize the various reflex points as being in a Christmas tree formation from the top of the body down. The reflexes mark various branches along the nerves' journey to the arms and legs – and, if absent or exaggerated, highlight areas where the fault may be localized.

Patients often gasp at their knees flying up in the air when tapped with a tendon hammer ('at least that is working' is the universal comment), like they did as children when they tapped their knee. I remind young students not to express similar delight when they 'get' a reflex for the first time – very uncool in front of patients and hardly reassuring if they appear bemused by their own competence.

At the end of the motor examination, I run a key or orange stick firmly along the soles of the feet. You may recall that in chapter 1 Jenny's big toes springing upwards told me that she had suffered serious nerve damage. This is a reflex called the Babinski (or plantar) response and testing it is an integral part of the neurology exam. It's a peculiar-seeming thing to have done to you and I can only wonder what patients think when they come to a doctor complaining of visual problems or headaches and he or she asks them to take off their shoes and socks and proceeds to scrape their feet firmly. (I have learned to explain what I am doing in detail after a young woman asked many years ago whether I had a foot fetish.) When we are born our big toes go up when the sole of the foot is stroked. After a year or so, stroking the sole causes the big toe to bend downwards in keeping with the development of our nervous system. If the nervous system is damaged in certain areas later in life, as can be the case in MS and many other neurological conditions, the toe assumes the 'baby state' and goes up again when the sole is stroked. It is one of the most important signs in clinical neurology, in my view, and toes curling up are never a good thing for the patient.

Having completed the motor testing I then do the sensory exam to assess the wires running in the opposite direction – from the hands and feet to the brain. Two of the main tools used for this are a tuning fork and a tooth pick, asking patients whether they can feel the vibration of the tuning fork or the sting of the tooth pick as I work up from their feet to their head. There are two main sensory lines. These determine how we respond to the world around us and explain how we react to pain, to hot plates and even how we feel our feet touch the ground. Again the goal of the sensory examination is to ascertain whether the return journey is interrupted and, if so, to work out where the 'train' has been derailed.

Once the location of the problem has been established, we try to determine what caused it. To do this we perform scans of the location, like mechanics taking photographs when they survey the site of a train crash. Only when we have been able to diagnose the site of the damage can we begin to try to fix it.

Precisely what to tell patients, and when, about what their condition might be is a delicate process. Naturally enough, they are extremely eager to have an immediate and full picture of what's going on. Sometimes I'll explain how I might suspect a certain diagnosis, because I've seen it many times before. Aware that I could be wrong, I won't go into the intricate details while we're waiting for tests to be performed. This inevitably leaves the patient with the impression that I am hiding something from them. And in a sense I am – but not with malice. I'm trying to protect them from unnecessary anxiety, in case my initial suspected diagnosis is wrong. If I were to list all of the possibilities – everything that might be wrong, called the differential diagnosis – I could scare them witless. Worried patients tend to have a heightened awareness of a doctor's mood and tone, and any apparent furtiveness leaves them feeling vulnerable. Patients' fear that they are losing control is an important part of the interaction too, especially for men it seems to me, where a sense of emasculation can be at play. No one likes the idea that their fate is in another person's hands.

Apart from judging how much information to give patients, choosing the right words can also be a challenge. On the one hand, your patients need to understand that you know what you're doing. On the other, you must be careful not to overwhelm them with jargon. There is a line between trying to engender confidence in your abilities and sounding arrogant. Like most doctors, I have inadvertently crossed that line, of course. When you are trying to explain very complex things that you have been studying for many years, it can be hard to give people a clear picture of their diagnosis and your understanding of it in a single consultation.

So, in delivering news, I try to get the balance right with every patient. And I fail with regularity. For instance, I can explain how we are going to do tests to rule out serious illnesses, only to hear them outside on their mobile saying, 'He thinks I have cancer.' And if I remain vague, either because I need more information from test results or I am suspicious that something serious is going on and I want to be absolutely sure before breaking bad news, I will hear them telling friends, 'He hasn't a clue.'

James's father and grandfather had Huntington's disease, as had two of his three brothers. Huntington's is a hereditary brain disease that leads to abnormal writhing movements, called chorea, and then dementia. One of his brothers had taken his own life at forty-three years of age when his brain began to disintegrate and he could no longer dress himself. James was forty-six and had been referred because he had begun to get 'the shakes' when presenting at business meetings in recent months.

We shook hands and he sat down in front of me. He had nicked himself shaving that morning, and the third button on his shirt was undone. I asked him to describe his symptoms, and he did so in a detached way, seemingly only mildly perturbed by having to sit on his right hand during meetings. At times he felt he was unable to control it. I asked about stress; he held a fairly high-powered post that meant long hours and sleepless nights worrying about 'the bottom line'. He had three children, the eldest of whom was heading to college in the autumn. James had worked hard to provide for himself and his family and happily admitted to a fairly comfortable lifestyle.

I asked about his family history and he went through it dispassionately; obviously he had always been keenly aware of Huntington's and its symptoms. Throughout the conversation he would intermittently rotate an arm in a very subtle but definite writhing movement (as we all do when scratching an itch and don't want to draw attention to the fact), or his leg would jerk forward very slightly from the chair he was sitting in.

I asked how long he had had these shakes.

'About a year or so, but they haven't bothered me that much till recently.'

'And has your wife noticed anything?'

'I'm not sure if she has or not. I don't think so. She hasn't said anything.'

I was fairly certain that James's wife had noticed, but exploring the extent of a patient's denial is worthwhile; I need to know how best to deliver bad news.

'Well, what do you think it could be?' I asked.

'You're the doctor,' he said, smiling. 'Just as long as it's not what my dad and brothers had, I'll be able to deal with it.'

Huntington's can come on at a variety of ages, and at forty-six, James thought the family disease had passed him by. It is a particularly cruel condition because it is inherited, but the chances of the children of a parent with the disease inheriting the genes is 50 per cent. A very accurate test can confirm whether you have the relevant genes; if you do, you will get the disease, but with what symptoms, or at what age, we can't be certain. James's brothers had developed symptoms in their early twenties, so James had reasoned that he was now too old to have inherited 'the family curse', as he called it. If he did, his three children would have a 50 per cent chance of getting it themselves. This can be the hardest part of a diagnosis for parents; the guilt they carry with them can be as hard to bear as the physical suffering of Huntington's and other genetic disorders. Symptoms typically start with unusual shaking and evolve into squirming movements. Eventually, it leads to dementia.

After talking to James for a few minutes, I had no doubt that he had the condition, but his denial was so deeply ingrained, I knew that the diagnosis would be particularly traumatic for him. You try to be straight with people without being too harsh, but there are occasions when dancing around what is self-evident can be unnecessarily cruel. I told James that I thought he might have the disease, but that other conditions could mimic Huntington's, so I would look for those too.

I arranged a variety of blood tests and a brain scan in the hope we could uncover an alternative diagnosis with a less grim prognosis, but I knew it wasn't to be. Doctors get scared of a terminal diagnosis too and I needed some time to come to terms with having to condemn him to the disease he'd always dreaded, and having to inflict panic on his wife and children. The family history was telling us what was staring him in the face. He signed the consent form for the genetic tests after I had explained the implications of a positive result.

'I think you are wrong on this one,' he said. He was still smiling, but less convincingly now. I hoped he was right.

A few weeks later he returned and a different personality stood before me. Gone was the jocular, confident businessman of a few weeks previously. He looked pale and drawn. He had discussed it with his wife and they had hardly slept with the worry waiting for the test result. They came together for this appointment and looked at me with desperation. They both knew there was to be no reprieve.

They cried as they held each other, and I promised meekly to see them again soon to go through things further when they had had time to gather their thoughts. At times like that there is nothing you can do other than to say you are sorry to be giving the news. I sat there, shell-shocked myself, as they left the room. After a few minutes the clinic nurse peered around the corner of the open door. 'The patients outside are getting restless,' she said. I scanned the next chart, stood up and went to the waiting room.

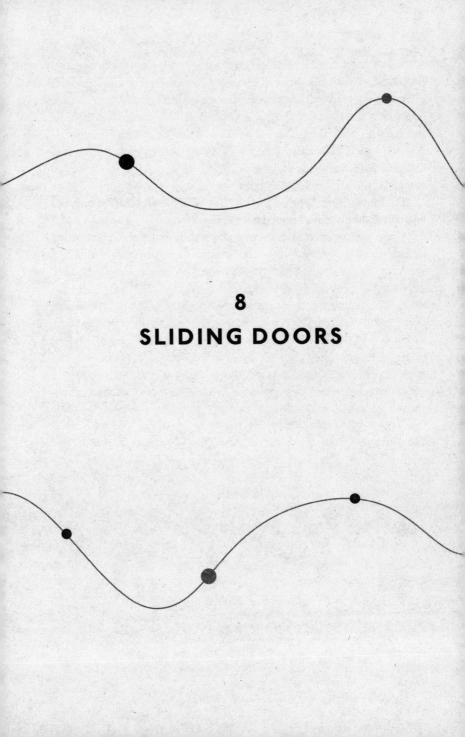

8

SLIDING DOORS

I was on call one evening as a senior house officer and met a lovely elderly lady who told me she was from Galway. When I told her my name, her face lit up and she proceeded to tell me a story about my grandfather, Seán Tubridy, who hailed from Oranmore. He had qualified as a young doctor in Galway, and was training to be a GP. He wanted to make some extra money, and successfully applied for a post in the remote coastal area of Connemara called Beal an Daingean, where the senior GP was about to go on his annual holidays and needed cover.

Seán arrived the night before he was due to start and was going through the handover of his duties with the GP when a call came looking for *an dochtuir* from one of the Irish-speaking islands nearby. I can only imagine his excitement – he'd have had little chance of 'home visits' by boat until now – but the local doctor said he'd take the call himself to 'clear the slate' for Seán. The senior GP set out with some local boatmen in a currach, a small rickety boat made in the traditional way, with animal skins stretched over a wooden frame. It was a rough night at sea and none of them made it back. Their bodies subsequently washed up on the mainland.

This is our genealogical 'sliding doors' moment. If my grandfather had been on that boat, my father would never have existed and I and my siblings would never have existed. I had never heard this story before. We've since verified it and it has stayed with our family ever since. The element of chance in all of our existences is both freakish and extraordinary. Seán went on to be a well-known GP in the Galway area and eventually was elected to the Dáil to represent the people of Galway.

Years later, another elderly patient mentioned the 'Tubridy stones' in her area of Connemara.

'What are they?' I asked innocently.

'Oh, don't you know?' she asked conspiratorially. 'Your grandfather would go on his house visits to very remote areas of the countryside. Most of our families had little or no money, so he would be paid with a meal and a drink or two.' She smiled. 'There was no such thing as electricity or street lighting at that time. There might have been the odd occasion when he was given' – so generous were her words – 'a bit too much to drink, so we would paint the stones in the road white to help guide him on his way!'

'Are you saying he was a drunk, then?' I asked.

'Not at all,' she said. 'That was the way of things back then.'

My grandfather died aged forty-two, apparently from a heart attack. Since hearing about the events of his first locum I have sometimes wondered if the trauma of his near miss affected him psychologically and whether he felt guilty about surviving when others perished. Maybe his premature death was hastened by the stress of surviving and too many drinks.

My father practised psychiatry for many years in Dublin. His speciality was helping people with alcoholism. I always wondered whether he chose, subliminally or otherwise, to treat alcoholics because of the stories about his father, who died when my father was three years old.

When we were younger, my siblings and I would go along with my father and our excitable Irish red setter on his weekend hospital visits where he did his rounds. It gave my mother a precious break for a few hours from the havoc created by five young children. He would park in the hospital car park and we would run wild in the grounds. We would gather pine cones in St Gabriel's or St John of God's for burning in our fire in the living room that evening, and the dog would chase whatever unfortunate birds were resting in the otherwise tranquil surrounds. Not infrequently, a janitor, nun or priest would come out to investigate the commotion being caused by these feral children and their mad dog. It is funny now to think of my poor dad going into the austere surrounds of the psychiatric wards, switching from parent to doctor mode, while we ran riot outdoors.

Occasionally, it wasn't so austere on the ward, however. Much later, I once witnessed mayhem on the locked unit of one of the hospitals in which he worked, and I thought how jarring it must have been, having to switch from the domesticity of children and a dog on a Saturday morning outing to the seriousness and desperation of the patients he was visiting. He would return to the small car exhausted and light up the first of many cigarettes, the five children and the red setter be damned, like a scene out of *Mad Men*.

In the days before mobile phones and the internet we had a single house phone and it is funny to recall the excitement the loud ringing in the hall would generate. We had to go ex-directory after a series of late-night calls from a few of his patients who had fallen off the wagon and were angry – at their own failure, at the doctor who had failed them – and indulging in the ultimate 'drunk dial'. The phone ringing was such a big deal that we would all wake to the racket. I knew how deeply it upset him and he would just be a bit quieter the next morning but life would go on as usual for us.

In the 1970s and 1980s psychiatry underwent some seismic changes and our father was sometimes described as 'old school' by the trainees I'd later meet – a back-handed compliment, perhaps, but his philosophy was a simple and straightforward one: listen, listen and listen some more. The film *One Flew Over the Cuckoo's Nest* became part of the social vernacular when it came out in the mid-1970s. Electroconvulsive therapy, popularly referred to as electric shock therapy, for people with depression so severe that anti-depressant drugs could not help them, was in relatively common use in psychiatric hospitals throughout the world, and Ireland was no exception. The changes wrought upon the Jack Nicholson character, 'Randle McMurphy', in the film sent a shiver down the spine of most audiences, and scared the world at large as to what could happen in 'the loony bin'. And any nurse who was anything less than sweetness and light every hour of every shift was cruelly dubbed 'Nurse Ratched' after the heartless nurse in the film.

My dad was involved in administering electroconvulsive therapy many times, he told me. Although it could seem cruel and violent, he assured me it was a far more controlled procedure than it was depicted in the movies, and some of his patients who had suffered with intractable depression for years had only gained respite by receiving ECT.

My father hated being asked about his work when out socially, in part I think because of how psychiatrists were perceived. Psychiatrists, he would say, instantly provoked fears in many that they might be analysing you even in everyday situations, so it must have been socially tricky at times. I know from some of my own interactions socially that some people think neurologists do the same thing, so I would be very surprised if psychiatrists did not still suffer the same stereotyping as my father even today. Then there was the stigma surrounding mental illness itself. How awkward it must have been socially in less open times when psychiatric illness and mental health in general were rather taboo subjects, seen as frailties of the mind (as they were), but also somehow the sufferer's own fault.

I have been lucky to have met many of my dad's former patients, or relatives of his patients, who very kindly have spoken highly of him. They tell me tales of how he saved their lives, their parents' lives or their marriages. I have met many of the doctors who trained under his supervision at one stage or another of their careers and, though hardly impartial, they tell me how much they learned from him and how much they admired his methods and the way he approached patients.

It is always lovely to hear nice things about your father. Of course, I don't hear from doctors who disagreed with how he went about things. It's nicer this way, but it would be foolish to convince yourself that all was rosy throughout the career of any doctor – particularly if you're trying to learn from it as a doctor yourself. I have met psychiatric in-patients who were treated by my father and his colleagues years before and still required treatment. Some, still sick, who realized that I was his son have vented about his shortcomings as a doctor. Even knowing how unwell they are it can be upsetting – to see them still unwell, knowing that my father must have done his best, and to be reminded that even our best efforts are not always enough.

As I grow older I am more sensitive to the vagaries of the doctor–patient interaction and appreciate the joys of a successful consultation, one during which you feel that you and the patient have communicated well, and hopefully you have affected the patient's life for the better. I also have had to accept the fact that no doctor can hope to get on well with all the people they encounter and with some there will never be a meeting of minds.

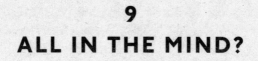

9
ALL IN THE MIND?

Jessica was a little late and somewhat flustered arriving into the Melbourne neurology clinic where I was working. Though she was Australian she reminded me of the English actor Helena Bonham Carter in her offbeat mannerisms and vintage clothing. I met her only once but she certainly made an impression. She was thirty-two and had become fixated with the idea there was something wrong with her right hand – her dominant hand – and asked her GP to refer her to a neurologist.

Once she appeared more settled she explained that the problem had evolved gradually. She liked to paint but had noticed that the strength in her right hand had diminished. Now and again when working at her easel she found it hard to reach the top of the large canvasses she worked with and had even taken to trying to paint with her left hand at times. Despite this deficit she had tried to ignore the problem but it had been getting progressively worse since the preceding December. That was more than six months earlier, so I asked why it had taken her so long to seek help. After a pause, and a fleeting glance to her left, she said she was not sure why but she just did not think it was anything serious.

I made the usual inquiries about her overall health, lifestyle and previous medical problems but there was nothing revealing. I asked whether there was any family history of neurological problems like MS, Parkinson's disease or motor neuron disease and she went quiet.

'I don't know,' she whispered. 'I haven't seen my family for nearly six months.'

At times like this I feel very intrusive and am never sure whether probing further into such family troubles will create more problems than solutions. I am very close to my family and struggle to understand the reasons why families fall apart and how people cope with the isolation from those who have known them best in their life. It is not uncommon, however, to see people like Jessica who have lost contact with parents and siblings, maybe for years, and sometimes they cannot even remember the original reasons for the rupture – or don't want to tell me.

I asked Jessica if she wanted to talk about it and she paused again.

Her gaze appeared to flit once more to her left side before returning to look me in the eye.

'No, Doctor, I would rather not go there.'

I examined her carefully and could find nothing wrong. The tone, power and co-ordination of her right hand appeared normal. All of the reflexes were present on her right side and equal to those on her left. I checked her ability to sense touch and gentle pain but again, all was intact. In a young woman like Jessica a neurologist would almost always want to exclude multiple sclerosis but there was nothing to indicate such a diagnosis. I asked what she had googled before coming to see me.

'I don't use the internet, Doctor. Never took to it.'

I found this astounding but strangely credible given her unusual affect during our conversation. For the third time I registered her looking to her left, in the direction of her left hand, which appeared to twitch intermittently as she gazed at it.

'Jessica, can I ask you if there's some reason you look towards your left from time to time?'

She flinched.

'I don't know what you're talking about. You're reading too much into things.'

'I wonder if you have some stress in your life at present. Sometimes – not always – when we can't find the cause of a symptom, it can be a sign of stress.'

Once again she looked towards her left hand, this time blushing slightly.

'No, no. I'm not under any stress. Well, there's the family situation, but I've made my peace with that.'

I backed off; I was pushing her too hard. I said I would like to arrange some blood tests and an MRI, but reassured her that I had not found anything untoward and was just making sure I wasn't missing anything.

'How much will they cost?' she asked.

'Oh, this is free. This is what we pay our taxes for,' I said.

She looked towards her left hand, which she raised to her left ear, and mimicked someone talking. I watched, mesmerized, and waited for an explanation, but none was forthcoming.

'I have to ask, Jessica, what is going on? What are you doing with your hand?'

'I'm just asking it for advice as to whether or not I should go ahead with your tests.'

She stood to put her jacket on and her hand rose to 'speak' to her again.

'What do you mean, Jessica? Is your hand talking to you?'

'No, Doctor, this' – she raised her left hand once more – 'is my angel.'

I persuaded her to sit down and explain. She told me that for the last six months her left hand had taken on a life of its own and had become her guardian angel that advised her on all aspects of her life.

She seemed perfectly sane in every other respect so I wondered how or why this odd behaviour had started. 'Has anything happened in the last year to upset you?'

She started to cry and caressed her left hand with her right. Her estranged father had turned up the previous Christmas Eve after many years abroad and there had been an almighty family row over the holiday period. Around New Year's Eve she started to believe her left hand was talking to her and guiding her through the troubled period. Far from finding this weird she took great comfort in her new-found angel and, knowing she had 'someone' she could rely on, was actually less anxious. This had become a fixed delusion and was causing her to act strangely, but it was not doing her any harm.

It did not take much on my part, other than holding up a mirror, for Jessica to see that the unresolved family feud had led to her current plight. She refused my offers to arrange counselling, and although she agreed to the tests I planned, she never turned up for the appointments. This happens more frequently than one might think, and I often find out later that people were afraid of what the tests might reveal.

I didn't see Jessica again before I left Melbourne but think of her from time to time and wonder what became of her. Do people like Jessica take a dislike to anyone who points out what is obviously a psychological problem? Can it be that when someone like Jessica is faced with the truth, problems such as hers gradually resolve themselves? Or perhaps she concluded she was content as she was and didn't want any more interference. Who knows, but there is only so much one can do. Doctors can feel a sense of failure in cases like Jessica's, but, when teaching medical students, I share Jessica's story to point out our limitations.

Debbie had had a similar problem when I met her in London in the late nineties. Her left hand had started to take on a life of its own one January. The difference between her and Jessica was that Debbie then started to have trouble walking as well and arrived at the clinic on crutches. She had a husband and two young children but came alone to her appointment. She had great family support, she assured me, and told me her family life was a very happy one.

Incredibly friendly and apparently open and sincere, Debbie was instantly likeable. I was taken aback, however, when, with much encouragement to get her to move her arms and legs, I could not find a clear-cut neurological problem. I was pleasantly surprised for her, as my initial – wrong – impression when she struggled in the door was that this was not going to turn out well.

I told her the good news, adding that in case I was wrong once more, I would look for the usual neurological suspects that can sometimes fool us. But I reassured her that I did not expect to find anything serious.

Her mood turned instantly and her sunny demeanour was replaced by a glare.

'How dare you say there is nothing wrong with me; what do you know anyway?' she said.

I was gobsmacked by this rapid change and tried to explain again that I was only glad for her that I had found nothing on my examination that might point to conditions like MS or MND but that I would be making doubly certain with the tests I had planned.

Throughout this very uncomfortable exchange Debbie's left hand had stopped rising in the air and it dawned on me (rather slowly, I admit) that this was what we describe as a functional neurological disorder. It was 'real' in that Debbie was displaying the symptoms she was presenting with, and that they originated in her brain, but there was nothing structurally wrong with her brain or nervous system. In times past we might have labelled Debbie's symptoms as 'psychosomatic'. We no longer do. The word is freighted with a level of judgement that we try to avoid. Frankly, it's not our business to judge people – there may be good reasons for a patient presenting with neurological symptoms that aren't real in the sense of arising from a genuine neurological problem. Instead, we try to find a way of helping them.

Giving Debbie vague explanations for her symptoms was not going to satisfy her or indeed facilitate her recovery. So I tried a different approach and spoke optimistically about how a problem like this was treatable and how, in due course, and with physical and perhaps some cognitive behavioural therapy, she could expect a return to normality, including going back to work.

'If you think I'll ever be well enough to go back to work then you haven't a clue what you're doing,' she shouted.

She was only twenty-eight years of age and had not worked for five years because of her disability. She was living on benefits. Surely, I said, she'd feel much better by regaining her self-confidence and becoming an active member of society again? I was wrong for the third time in quick succession.

'You can go fuck yourself, you prick!' she said and stormed out of the room.

I paused for a minute and took a few deep breaths to regain my composure. I stood to call the next patient and asked the clinic nurse to chase after Debbie as she had forgotten her crutches.

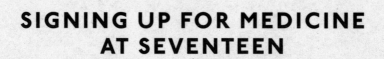

10

SIGNING UP FOR MEDICINE AT SEVENTEEN

It was only later in life that I truly considered how my father's medical speciality might have influenced who he was. A kind and patient man, he didn't have much time for academia and just spoke frankly to thousands of patients over his thirty or more years as a doctor. He was a great listener and always advised us to try to hold back from rushing to judge people. (I am not sure how successful that lesson was!) He was generally quiet and had a very droll, sometimes acerbic, sense of humour.

Unlike his children, he had been a great sportsman. He played as a flanker on his school's rugby team and won a senior cup medal in 1954 playing against a famous Belvedere team graced by Tony O'Reilly, who later played for Ireland and the Lions. Although Dad rarely mentioned it, his rugby friends from years previously would delight in regaling me with the stories of how our father stopped 'O'Reilly' winning a coveted Schools' Cup medal. He played water polo to a high level, but we never heard of this until a few years later. He was a good sailor, but I never saw him near a boat. Most of his children turned out to be borderline hydrophobic. When I asked him about these pursuits he would just shrug and say 'self-praise is no praise'.

He attended our awful attempts at rugby, soccer, hockey and whatever was our sport *du jour* without complaint. He would stand on the sidelines of our little sporting lives, always smoking discreetly, regardless of the rain and wind. He encouraged our every transient interest in music (an old piano lasted about six months), art, genealogy and even orienteering at one point. Now I think how he must have worried as he saw young men and women at the same ages as his own children succumb to alcohol, drugs or, worse still, suicide.

When I mentioned that I was thinking of applying to medical school he seemed pleased in his understated way.

'Are you sure that is what you want?' he asked. Detecting some reservation on his part, I asked him whether or not he thought it was a good idea.

'It is a great thing to do,' he said, 'but it is a very long road.'

I knew it meant six years in medical school before you were qualified, but I did not quite appreciate, until he explained the process to me, how many years after you were able to call yourself 'Doctor' it was until you actually felt like a proper doctor. He explained that the first post upon qualification was a year as an intern – the lowest rung on the ladder. Then you became a senior house officer for two or three years, in which time you experienced many aspects of medicine before considering a longer-term speciality. Once decided, you would spend five to ten years as a registrar training to be a consultant. During that latter time you would have to spend many years abroad, away from your friends and family, with few opportunities in those days to travel home (due to the expense of air travel and the hours that you would be working). None of this was enough to put me off.

I had not considered medicine seriously until my latter years in school. I was a fairly bright child, I believe, but went off the rails a bit in my early and mid-teens. I started to hang out with slightly older kids in the local area and schoolwork quickly fell down my list of priorities as I pathetically tried to keep up with my socially more mature peer group. At around fourteen I started to drink and smoke. My schoolwork suffered as a result of my social proclivities, and I lost interest in many of the subjects we were studying, and in school in general. I liked history and Latin but had no particular penchant for chemistry and biology, and physics was completely alien to me. I was, and still am, pretty terrible at all things mathematical. I love things that appear logical and follow a defined path yet, paradoxically, could not grasp maths or physics. I worked very hard at the former so as not to face what I felt was the failure of dropping to the lower-level maths class, but I was really not able for it. My parents paid for extra tuition and I did my best, but my studies in other subjects suffered as a result of the inordinate time I had to put in to try (and fail) to master algebra and trigonometry.

I considered journalism, social work and law as alternative career options, but once I got my act together in my last two years at school I realized medicine was within my grasp. I also began to get the idea it was exactly what I wanted, but, fearful of not getting the points, I played down my ambitions in front of my friends and my family until my grades started to improve.

It was around this time that my parents' marriage came to an end. It

was very upsetting for everyone, not least because of the social embarrassment that separated families suffered in early-1980s Ireland. It was
still an unusual event in those years and, while undoubtedly the best
thing for all concerned in the long run, it made us feel somewhat 'other'
for a few years. As a result, my siblings and I are incredibly close and
have all made our own ways fairly independently since our teenage
years. It is remarkable now to reflect on how my parents, like so many
of their generation, married and settled down so young. They were
both very loving in their own ways, but they were such different personalities that, in hindsight, parting seemed inevitable.

Being of an age when I was allowed to decide which parent to live
with, I opted to move in with my dad. I am not sure he wanted this (he
did not want to separate me from my siblings), but I was nothing if not
persistent.

My confidence that I could get the points for medicine grew in my
penultimate year at school when I started to get decent results in my
term exams for the first time since I was about twelve years old. After a
few humiliating evenings left standing outside whatever pubs or clubs
my older friends were now frequenting, I became socially isolated for
a while. Although I was sad to feel excluded, in retrospect it was the
making of me. With little in terms of distractions I realized I might as
well do some work and it began to pay off quite quickly. And that was
when I finally broached doing medicine with my parents.

Having spent most of her adult life married to a doctor, Mum understood the ups and downs of a life in medicine, but she respected my
own judgement about whether it would be a fit for me. In a different
way, Dad was also neutral on the matter. Having pointed out the long
road to becoming a doctor, he neither encouraged nor discouraged my
decision to apply for medicine. I suspect now that he didn't want to
feel responsible for my career decisions – especially one made at such
a young age that is more or less what you will do for the rest of your
life. Of course, from the perspective of a seventeen-year-old, the idea of
a life-long commitment to anything is impossible to contemplate. He
was still a relatively young man at that point, but had been a consultant
for about ten years. He had five children and a thriving practice, but I
recognize now that even ten years in the same emotionally arduous

job can take its toll. Maybe he was afraid I might not be able to manage what he sometimes laboured to cope with. I wish we had discussed it in a more in-depth way and regret the conversations we didn't have. I never even asked him why he became a doctor. In any case, at the age I was making the life-altering decision to become a doctor, the emotional intelligence gap between us was probably too wide for me to comprehend even if he had explained the truth about (his and later, my) life in medicine.

My father's reality check notwithstanding, I still had romantic notions of helping people as well as a sense of curiosity about how the body worked. By my final year in school I decided I would apply for medical school and worked almost obsessively to achieve that goal. I would get up early to get in an hour's study before school. I would work hard for hours each evening and spend many more hours studying alone at weekends. Years later my poor sisters and brothers, who would stay over at the weekends, took great pleasure in telling me precisely what a pain in the ass I was back then. They would spend their precious weekends with our father whispering around the house, because I needed silence to study. I was a dreadful brother at that stage, as I felt it was somehow me against the world and nothing was going to get in the way of my studies.

When I started medical school the following September, I still looked like a child. On my first day my father dropped me to the top of Grafton Street to walk the last hundred yards to the Royal College of Surgeons. He was pleased as Punch, I think, and probably a wee bit envious as, though he knew better than most the hard work that lay ahead, he also knew about the fun the next six years would entail. He would tell me about his college days only sporadically, after we had had a few pints.

We lived together, like two bachelors, for the entire period of my medical school years. For those six years I became detached from my siblings and my mother to some extent, only to recover our friendships as I got to the end of my training. In the meantime I found my new family among my medical student friends. Such is the intensity of the bonds formed in medical school when, at only seventeen or eighteen years of age, you spend most of your waking hours in each other's company both at work and at play. I had friends at school and have met new friends since I qualified, but few friendships are as deep as those with my medical school friends.

As I tried to come to terms with my parents' separation and the surreal nature of seeing my siblings at weekends as they stayed over, my new medical student friends never made any issue of their split. We would work in study groups in my dad's small house and sit around for hours pretending to work together, but mostly I just recall the fun of it all. Though I still lived at home I had far more freedom than my peers and took full advantage of it, to the enduring aggravation of my poor father. I went a little wild once more and it amazes me still how I managed to pass the early exams given the amount of time I spent in the various pubs and clubs around the College of Surgeons.

He would cook a dinner each evening for the two of us, and every Saturday morning he would fume when I had gone straight to the pub from college and had never let him know I would not be home to share it with him. 'There is half a chicken in the oven,' he would remark casually the next morning, relishing my pain in my hungover state.

Dad seemed to like my friends being around and we spent many long nights drinking beer with him. He was getting used to his own new-found sense of freedom as well as, I imagine, a sense of isolation. I shudder at my insensitivity to the emotional trauma he must have been feeling, coming to terms with the ending of a more than twenty-year marriage and facing into middle age alone. You become more aware of such things when you hit middle age yourself. My world then was all about me. How selfish I was, but he was so kind in allowing me to get on with my life and rarely interceded.

In the first few years in particular we would go out together at least once a week and I would talk at length about the events of that week. Although he might not have been able to help much directly with my studies, as I progressed through my early college years I got to know him more as an older friend. He became important as a counsellor to help me through periods of doubt. He listened and laughed along with what I assume were now our common experiences (for instance, he recognized all too well the clammy feeling of walking into an anatomy room and first sighting a cadaver). He never pretended it was easy but would point out the pros more than the cons at that stage. As we both got older I understood that in my fledgling days in medicine – as a student and junior doctor – he was at the peak of his career and still very interested in the job.

It was not always one-way traffic and, as I was the only one around all of the time, he would confide in me at times about the trials and tribulations of his own medical life. He would tell stories of success and, more often, terrible tales of the failures. He spoke about how he felt about some of his (unnamed, of course) patients. I would hear through the grapevine of fellow medical students who were finding things hard and had resorted to drugs or alcohol to such a level of dependence that they had ended up under his care. I asked him about this a couple of times but he would never discuss any individuals and only dealt with generic examples – perhaps using these as a subtle way of trying to keep his sometimes wayward son on the straight and narrow.

As a young student, occasionally I went with him on his weekend rounds and was transfixed by the patients wandering forlornly around the wards who appeared to be in some sort of fog-like state but would turn slowly and smile when he greeted them. He saw how curious I was about medicine and I always hope it imbued in him a sense of renewed enthusiasm in his own work. It was odd to realize how much about the medicine I was learning he, a long-qualified doctor, did not know. I asked him about my undergraduate subjects like biochemistry and physiology a few times and he would mutter under his breath something along the lines of how little these things mattered when someone was sitting in front of you with their life falling apart. I did not understand until much later in life how right he was.

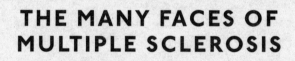

11

THE MANY FACES OF
MULTIPLE SCLEROSIS

About four times a week I tell people that they have MS. It never gets easier giving a patient bad news, and just when I think I have got the approach right – being as positive but honest as I can be – that is the moment I might get it wrong. It can be tricky to get the phrasing right. A poor choice of words will stay with them for ever. A kind word will give them something to rake over optimistically later, but it may be misleading. And each individual's interpretation of the same explanation is different.

It is important not to draw out the conversation, as it can add to the stress. I sometimes wonder whether the people in front of me hear anything until I say whether they have whatever disease they've been dreading or not; they often seem to tune out of the conversation until we get to the bottom line.

MS may present with something dramatic, like loss of vision, or a sudden problem walking, talking or swallowing, all of which are extremely alarming. But it can also present in a way that seems more benign, like pins and needles in an arm or leg. The majority of cases begin with a single neurological episode. When meeting a patient who has symptoms that suggest MS, the history is as important as the MRI scan in understanding how their MS is manifesting. I tailor some of the questions to try to identify previous attacks, as they may have occurred many years previously, and were then discounted by the patient as being something else. It's understandable, as the attacks, at least initially, tend to be self-limiting – many people recover fully without any medical intervention in as little as a few weeks. Some people might experience what feels like an electric shock going down their arms and legs whenever they bend their neck forward. Patients say that they thought they had a crick in their neck, or they had had a sports injury around the same time, so they had rested and it had gone away.

Some people are lucky and have a single episode that looks like MS, but in fact isn't, and they never have another episode again. Indeed, there are people who have lived with an MS diagnosis for forty years or more who don't have MS at all. They were diagnosed at a time when the diagnostic tools available were not as precise as they are now and there seemed to be no other explanation for their neurological symptoms. Other people have a first episode and go on to have recurrences throughout their lives. They recover between attacks (remission), and then feel safe for a short period before it strikes again (relapse).

We do not know what causes MS exactly, but we think it is a disorder of the immune system that affects some who may be genetically predisposed to the condition. You could say that about a lot of illnesses, like arthritis and inflammatory bowel disease, so it is a bit of a catch-all explanation for the many medical conditions for which we still do not know the exact cause, especially in neurology.

Anita had enjoyed medical school, and when she qualified she found working as an intern exhilarating. She didn't mind the long hours or the late nights. She could handle the sleeplessness and the middle-of-the-night bleeps. Her excitement about what might happen on each shift left her practically euphoric, though she was anxious about making mistakes.

Late one night, she was called to a young man with cancer. He was in the terminal stages, and had been extremely sick from the failing attempts at treatment. Anita tried to console the emaciated patient, who could not stop vomiting, and she reflected afterwards that here was a man a few years older than her who wouldn't be alive at the end of the year. She moved on to the next ward to answer the next bleep.

This time, she rewrote the drug chart of an elderly woman. It could have been left until the morning, but seeing as she was up already, she thought she'd get on with it. As she transcribed the list of the woman's medication from the chart to the fresh file, she squinted to read the names of the drugs. She turned on the bedside light, but still found it a strain picking out the words on the pages. She was exhausted, she reasoned, and decided to abandon her efforts. It could wait until morning. She made her way back to the doctors' residence, and lay down for a rest. When she was called an hour or so later, she couldn't make out the number on her pager, and she now became conscious of a dull ache in her right eye. When she looked around the dimly lit room her eye hurt, and she realized quickly that she could hardly see anything. She covered her sore right eye, and found she could see out of the left, but when she covered her left eye she was almost blind.

Anita was one of my favourite undergraduate students. She was witty and very intelligent, and didn't take herself too seriously. She was empathetic towards patients, and had a good sense of human nature. When she sat with me in clinics, we would analyse the social aspects of each case as much as the neurological problems, and she was precociously astute in her assessments of people and the influence of their environments.

I see at least five junior doctors a year who worry that they have developed neurological problems, and on only two occasions in more than twenty years has it ever been anything serious. Most of them have been recently exposed to a neurology patient and wonder whether their symptoms – headaches, fatigue or a muscle twitching – signify that they too have developed a terrible neurological condition. A combination of a little knowledge, chronic sleeplessness and baseline anxiety is generally the cause, and it's perfectly understandable.

But when Anita called in to me in the clinic the next morning, it was clear straight away that something was seriously wrong. She cried throughout the examination, as she had spent the last two hours googling her symptoms (a case of 'physician, do not heal thyself') and had spent enough time with me in our clinics to know that painful loss of vision in one eye in a young woman was most likely inflammation of her optic nerve (optic neuritis) – commonly one of the first signs of MS. I could not reassure her; the examination proved she was right. She had reduced appreciation of colour and limited central vision. The rest of her examination was normal, so I arranged an MRI scan for later that day. We gave Anita a course of intravenous steroids, and she recovered her vision over the next few weeks.

The MRI scan showed the ominous white spots that tend, in people with MS, to gather around what looks like the shoreline of the lakes of fluid in the brain, the ventricles. The clusters of white spots emanate from the area of the brain that connects the right and left hemispheres in a pattern known as Dawson's fingers – when viewed in profile on a scan they look like a bright Mohican haircut on the inside of the brain.

These white-spot areas represent various types of injury to the nerves (or wiring) of the brain and spinal cord. In the early stages of MS, the wires can lose some of their insulation in a process called demyelination; the wire isn't broken, but conducts less efficiently than before. It's like a dodgy lamp: the light works when you switch it on, but may flicker a little. Later in the disease more and more of the insulation, or myelin, can be affected and the light flickers more often. Eventually, the wire itself becomes damaged and the light may hardly function at all. So these white spots are areas of 'high signal' on the MRI scans that represent plaques in the brain where the sheath protecting the nerves has become inflamed and usually indicate MS.

I had sent her for other tests looking for conditions that can mimic MS, but to no avail. Anita had, as of now, a mild form of relapsing remitting MS. We set up other tests to confirm the diagnosis, which they did, and I knew Anita would never be the same bubbly, enthusiastic young woman ever again.

Sitting in front of Anita and her distraught parents a few weeks later to deliver the diagnosis I thought of Jenny – the young woman from chapter 1 who was my first MS patient. She often comes to mind when I am delivering a new diagnosis. Anita was twenty-four years old, and working seventy or more hours a week as a doctor, and planned on becoming a surgeon. But what would her future hold, with a diagnosis of MS hanging over her? Neither of her parents was a doctor, so unlike most parents, intuitively they deferred to their daughter. She already knew the diagnosis and had done her research, but regardless of who they are, it's not uncommon for patients to refuse to believe they have MS, because they feel so well, until they hear it from a neurologist. Anita nodded grimly when I gave her the diagnosis. Her father put his arm around her shoulder and her mother cried.

Anita said she wanted to start therapy straight away. She discussed her options pragmatically, but had made her decision. We agreed to treat her with one of the interferon injections that had become available as one of the first effective drugs for MS some years earlier. Interferon works to reduce possible future relapses by lessening the rogue response of the immune system that is thought to cause MS attacks.

For Anita, as for so many young people with MS, the question of what to do next ran deep. Had her ambition to be a surgeon been thwarted? As I had learned by now, it was not my role to judge but to try to help. What if she developed symptoms in the future while operating? What if she had no attacks for years, became a surgeon and only then developed symptoms that would prevent her doing the only job she had spent years training for? There are so many 'what ifs' and no definitive answers.

'I never thought, as I dreamed of becoming a doctor, that I would actually become a patient,' she said. My heart broke for her.

Patients managing a long-term disease have a lot to deal with, and Anita taught me so much about the insecurities that a neurological diagnosis like MS can instil. The interferon therapy caused her some side effects – flu-like symptoms after some of her early injections – and she felt run down while taking it. Interferons can cause depression in the first few months, but it can be hard to distinguish from the perfectly natural change in mood you might expect to see in a young, vibrant person who has suddenly been given a diagnosis of MS. Anita became increasingly timid, and I was sorry to see her lose her confidence.

Gradually Anita settled into a routine, giving herself the injections three nights a week. She said she had gorgeous moments when she was free of any thoughts of her dreaded condition, but no sooner was she enjoying life than she would be due another injection. It sounded like a form of emotional torture.

Our goal is to help our patients to resume their everyday routines and many people with MS live normal lives. Of course, the diagnosis never leaves them; they have to keep up with their medication, check-ups and therapies. Yes, the landscape of their lives will have changed, but what I often hear is simply, 'I just have to get on with it, don't I?' So, Anita would turn up for her appointments along with the 700 or so other people with MS who attended our clinics each year back then. There, she would see the worst cases, the people who don't respond to therapy, the people who are profoundly disabled by spasms and loss of muscle control. The sight of such patients stays with the more fortunate in the waiting room, and makes a greater impression than the majority breezing in and out of their annual reviews on their way back to their busy lives.

Each time I called Anita in, she'd wave and smile, but it would be less than five minutes before the tears would flow. Coming up to two years after her diagnosis, I started wondering whether the combination of injections and seeing me was doing more psychological damage than the actual MS. Her scans showed no progression in that time, and she had no attacks, so she continued her fledgling medical career.

Anita got more comfortable with the diagnosis and, with good news of no new white spots on consecutive scans, optimism began to creep in. Then, however, the scans showed a few new white spots. (This can happen even when someone has had no clinical attacks or relapses and suggests that the brain is being damaged even if there are no symptoms. It is another reminder of how little we know of the workings of the brain.) At this news, Anita admitted that, though she liked me personally, she hated seeing me around the hospital, particularly if she was feeling relatively well; no one likes to see the doctor who is a reminder of an illness that will never go away, and, unlike most, she had to go to work with hers.

A few years into her illness, and decades after the first wave of effective MS treatments, a new option became available that didn't need to be injected. Anita jumped at the chance to take a tablet instead of an injection, even if it meant doing so every day for the foreseeable future. Nothing is for ever in life, I reminded her – new, better and less intrusive therapies were being developed every couple of years.

Though easier and less upsetting for patients than injections, tablets bring their own problems. Everyone starts with the best of intentions, but research has shown that up to half of the people taking MS medications begin to miss taking them when they should and some stop altogether. Ironically, they can feel much better as a result – between the lack of side effects and the freedom from the daily reminder of MS – but stopping treatment puts them at risk of further attacks. With each attack comes the chance that someone won't recover, leaving them for ever with a blind eye or a weak leg, for example. In spite of the risks, it's difficult to persuade young people to think long term when they see their friends enjoying life to the full, free of the anxieties that constrain their lives. Some are frightened into a kind of apathy, and others cut loose completely with alcohol and illicit drugs, with an attitude of 'I'm going to die young anyway, so what's the point?'

Anita didn't go in for that, but was certainly much better psychologically on the new tablet for MS. Happily, there was no new activity on her scans for a further two years. She brought her non-doctor boyfriend along for one consult to hear me say how well she was, and to explain to him what I had been explaining to her about MS for years. She was clearly in love with him, and he with her. I was delighted for her, but my old fears about MS and relationships gnawed away. I asked him how he felt about Anita having MS (having asked her permission to do so in advance), and whether he had any questions of his own about the condition. His response surprised me for its levity and said more about them as a couple than how the disease had affected them, which was an answer in itself.

'We met in Coppers,' he said, laughing, referring to the legendary Dublin night club. 'She's great fun, and I'm in awe of her work as a doctor. I've never met someone I've admired so much. Sure, she looks after me more than I look after her.'

Anita beamed with pride.

'We're going to Australia for a year,' she said, 'and I've decided not to pursue surgery – but not because of this stupid MS. I just didn't like the long hours and the stress of it.'

When I next heard from her she was working in her new speciality. She emailed out of the blue one day to say she was doing well, and had married 'the boy from Coppers', as she called him. She asked what I thought about her having children.

In years gone by, when there were no treatments and no scans to monitor the condition, neurologists sometimes advised young women not to have children. Imagine what a terrible blow that was on top of a diagnosis of MS. Thankfully that has changed and, although it undoubtedly adds another layer of anxiety, most of the young women I see now have babies if they want to. Still, old stereotypes of the disease abound and are hard to shake. I recall one patient, Nicola, who was diagnosed with very mild MS in her late teens. I was thrilled when, years later, Nicola and her husband brought their baby boy to her appointment a few weeks after the delivery. She had had no problems with MS throughout her pregnancy, but was distraught because a midwife in the UK had suggested she be careful when holding her son because of, 'You know, the MS.' I am sure the midwife didn't mean to be cruel but the effect of such a remark on the sleep-deprived new mother was crushing in her moment of jubilation. After all, if an experienced medic could make such a clumsy remark, what must everyone else come out with?

As a neurologist my perspective on motherhood for young women with MS is quite practical. In addition to the joy of having children, the responsibilities they bring mean that people have less time to dwell on their MS. They also start to take their medication much more fastidiously, now that they have another reason to try to stay as well as they possibly can.

When she was diagnosed, Anita's attitude to motherhood had been 'I'm not having children and am going to concentrate on my career for as long as I am well.' So when I heard from her it gladdened me to learn that she had changed her mind. I said that she should not get pregnant while taking the medication but she could stop taking it while trying to conceive and throughout pregnancy. The medication is not risk-free and has the potential to damage a developing baby. Of course, there was a risk of an attack while she was off the medication, but ultimately this was a decision that only she could make. Given the excellent state of her health, I said she should go for it if she wanted to.

Within a year I got another email. Anita sent me a photograph of herself, the boy from Coppers and their two-month-old daughter on the beach in Sydney. She was keeping well, and enjoying both work and life. She talked of the future and coming home to Ireland. She even asked for a reference for a post that she planned to apply for in the coming months. Her confidence had returned. I am sure she still had dark moments, but now I could see that she could live, and live well, with this curse of a disease.

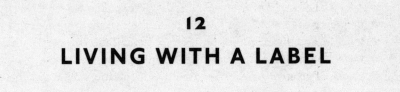

12

LIVING WITH A LABEL

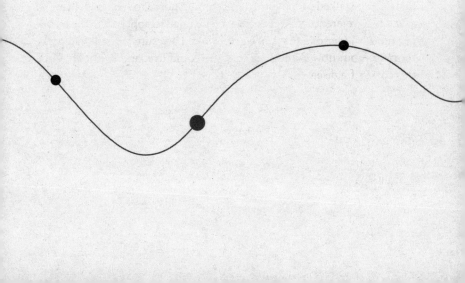

'Neurology? Why would you bother?' asked one of my senior colleagues, genuinely puzzled by my interest in the field, 'You'll be replaced by MRI scans soon enough.' He had a point. The introduction of magnetic resonance imaging scans gave insights into the brain that were almost unthinkable up to that point. For neurologists it was as mind-blowing as kids getting a new-generation computer game. But MRI studies, while undoubtedly an outstanding diagnostic tool that have transformed the work of neurologists and many other specialists, come with their own problems.

When I started training, MRI scanning was in its infancy, so even making a diagnosis of MS relied on carefully assessing the patient's symptoms and then a very detailed examination. Many times I saw consultants not even mention the possibility of MS to patients who had only suffered one or two intermittent attacks; in essence, the patient would go into an extended remission and we would adopt a 'wait and see' policy. The doctor would hope that the would-be patient didn't experience any more symptoms, and, if they didn't, would never hear from them again. They handled it this way mainly because there were no therapies on offer; as a result, the outcome for each patient was a question of luck rather than any medical intervention.

Nowadays someone who never had any MS symptoms might have an MRI scan – for a headache, say – and the scan picks up, incidentally, the clustered white spots that may indicate MS. This is particularly difficult for neurologists to deal with. We can't ignore the findings, but should we treat with anti-MS drugs someone who has never had any symptoms? Usually not, is the answer at the moment – although it depends on the case, and some neurologists do treat at this stage. Practice varies internationally and patient choice is also critically important.

We do, however, treat people who have had a single attack and whose MRI suggests that they will go on to develop MS in the future. So we now have a generation of mainly young people who have had only a single episode of neurological dysfunction and are otherwise perfectly well, but have started on a therapy because they are more likely than not going to develop MS and potential disability in the future – but not definitely.

It is emotionally fraught for the patients. How much information is too much? How much is not enough? Though a patient may go the rest of their lives symptom-free, they now have to live with the label of MS, which is a huge burden. When you try to make the discussion conversational and ask what they think themselves, not infrequently you will hear, 'Well, you're the doctor, you tell me.' Fair enough, I think, but, as with many illnesses of the brain, things are rarely black and white.

Most people who come to the clinic for the first time these days will have already made the diagnosis themselves online. As a result they are not only more informed – or misinformed – than the patients of the past, but, as a result, more anxious when we meet. They'll have come across the Lhermitte's phenomenon, the name for the sensation I described earlier – a feeling like an electric shock that can happen when someone bends their neck and then spreads down and makes the arms and legs feel tingly. This can be an early sign of MS and they will have resigned themselves to life in a wheelchair by the time they see the GP, let alone a neurologist.

At times, patients' online research can be extremely useful, as they have some basic knowledge about MS. But as often as not their anxiety muddies the water and I have to work out which symptoms are real and which have been picked up and assimilated – unwittingly – over the weeks or months the poor person has been waiting to be seen and trawling the internet.

Beyond the immediate reaction of stunned disbelief, even when a patient is expecting a diagnosis of MS, I can still never predict how someone will respond when they hear the words spoken out loud. Almost everyone cries. For some there may even be relief – since MS can come on insidiously, with vague symptoms of fatigue and non-specific complaints of one sort or another, when eventual investigations yield a diagnosis patients who felt they were going mad, or whose families had dismissed their worries, feel vindicated.

When it's a young person, initially parents tend to be more upset than the patient. With couples, the partner will reach for the patient's hand (for that is often how the person with the diagnosis is now seen, by themselves and those around them – no longer a person but a patient) and grimly seek reasons to remain upbeat. Unfortunately, the odd spouse will have over-googled and, in a well-meant bid to manage events, and oblivious to the emotional fall-out for their loved one, will start to focus on 'solutions'. This can be unthinkingly cruel – for instance, asking how long before their wife or husband will have to use a wheelchair, or how soon should they renovate the house to make it disability-friendly.

With the discovery of therapies that significantly reduce the risk of relapses (attacks), a diagnosis of MS is often not as dreadful as it once was and we approach many cases as very manageable. We can also treat many of the symptoms such as pain, leg spasms, and problems with bladder and bowel function. We work with physiotherapists, occupational therapists and speech therapists who further help to make living with the condition more bearable. However, not everyone responds to these therapies and some people still end up disabled and dependent. Still, it is vitally important at the outset, when the inevitable question arises – 'What next?' – that we can offer a range of options and, above all, hope for the future.

After a diagnosis the patient's world has been changed for ever. For a few weeks, the things that had once kept them up at night will pale into insignificance. The mortgage, work, their elderly parents; all become less pressing as they face the fact of their mortality. How will their spouse see them now? When they're exhausted after a hard day at work, will people respond by tilting their heads in sympathy? Never again will someone shake off the numb hand they wake up with without worrying they're having an attack that heralds the next phase of their condition.

Some people with MS report that their symptoms get worse in hot weather (a well-recognized complaint called Uhthoff's phenomenon), whereby a patient experiences a recurrence of previous symptoms while their body temperature is elevated. I always recall a young tennis fanatic with MS who played the game to a reasonably competitive level until he started to miss the ball to his right – but only after the fourth set. He gave up his favourite game as he worried he was 'making his MS worse' (this was not the case), just as some patients give up family sun holidays they always enjoyed. These are small ways that living with MS can sap the joy out of life, even when the condition isn't very far advanced; the effects can be very dispiriting – not just for patients, but for those around them too.

There is so much to ask and so much to tell in such a limited time when breaking the news of a diagnosis. We don't know with any certainty the course that MS will take in a given individual. The majority of people who develop MS have what's called a relapsing-remitting course: they suffer an attack, then recover, and then have another attack later. Many of these people will eventually stop recovering from attacks. Then the condition usually enters a slowly progressive phase, called secondary progressive MS, whereby the person gradually accumulates progressive disability, ending up possibly needing crutches or a wheelchair. A smaller subgroup of people get a type of MS that is, as yet, less treatable, called primary-progressive, which gets steadily worse without any remissions from the onset, and is stubbornly resistant to the therapies that can help the relapsing-remitting type.

Because doctors don't know the exact cause of MS, patients with the disease feel even more vulnerable. Doctors cannot accurately and honestly predict what someone with the label of MS will be like in a year, or two or ten. We can, with experience, look at a person and their scans and offer various therapies that will hopefully ameliorate the disease, but we can never be sure. I have sometimes told someone they are doing well, only to hear from them weeks or months later that they have had a serious attack. And I have privately feared the worst for a young man or woman who presents with what appears to be an aggressive form of MS, only to find the treatment working wonderfully.

I see people with relatively benign disease who had a single episode in the 1970s, another in the 1980s, and who are only very intermittently affected by the condition throughout their long lives. In fact, some people who have died of something else entirely have turned out to have had MS that was found only at their post-mortem; they never even knew they had it. Yet regardless of the wide spectrum of ways the disease can affect people, most of us have a fixed picture in our minds of the wheelchair and a life of dependence that will follow a diagnosis. Only when you've seen thousands of people with MS can you really appreciate how varied the condition can be. There is far more to it than the label might suggest to most people.

Regardless of the many medical therapies that have been developed over the last two decades, when discussing treatment for MS it is my experience that people are most likely to ask me first about changing their diet. It is as if in some way the diagnosis is their fault, which it most certainly is not.

Many come equipped with a list of potential cures for the disease. These tend to run in trends down the years. When I was in London in the late 1990s, a woman in the UK received a lot of publicity for her MS 'cure', a cocktail of vitamin B12, Coca-Cola and an anti-depressant. As with all such fads, it took a long time for this 'therapy' to fade from the popular imagination. Another belief that took hold was that mercury caused MS, and so people began to have all of their old dental fillings removed. And on they go. A few years ago, a surgeon in Italy treated his wife who had MS by dilating the veins in her neck. The theory, in essence, was that MS may be due to congestion of the veins; by dilating them, the 'drainage' system of the blood from the brain, and thus the condition itself, would be improved. Vulnerable patients were flocking to clinics across Continental Europe to have the expensive procedure. The publicity online was intense, the clamour was growing for it to become part of routine treatment for MS, and the treatment had to be rigorously investigated by neurologists. It was never definitively proven to work, and it too appears to be fading away.

Friends and families commonly ask about complementary or alternative therapies that can help. Cannabis is the main one. In a few studies cannabis has been shown to – possibly – alleviate the spasms some people with MS and other neurological conditions can develop. We have many proven drugs for such spasms and offer these, but there is something of the conspiracy theory about the non-use of cannabis – people seem to think the government is denying their loved ones the treatment they need or that doctors don't want to give the drug as they are in the pockets of 'Big Pharma'. A spray form of cannabis has been made legal in Ireland, but for reasons unclear we still cannot get it for our patients. My colleagues and I have tried unsuccessfully to source some, legally of course, for patients via Northern Ireland. As for doctors having an ulterior motive in protecting drug company interests, that doesn't hold up because the anti-spasm drugs we prescribe are mainly off patent, so there is a range of relatively cheap generic versions we can use.

I am not sure what harm a cannabis spray could do, though there isn't enough research yet to back up the myriad claims made for it. It is the current internet-fuelled panacea for all neurological ills, with claims of successful treatment of everything from Parkinson's disease to MS to back pain and headaches. 'Whatever works' is my mantra, but I am sure someone is making a lot of money out of a treatment that has yet to be proven.

Patients or the families of patients with severe MS regularly ask about stem-cell transplantation. Family members will offer to remortgage the house to pay for it, such is their desperation and eagerness to help. Stem-cell transplantation has shown serious promise for the future but it is still in its infancy in terms of treating most people with MS. I have yet to see a successful outcome from stem-cell therapies in private clinics abroad that are advertised on the internet. I have advised many people not to travel for these prohibitively expensive treatments; procedures can cost up to €80,000. Often they and those who love them will mount high-profile fund-raising drives to pay for their trip. Inevitably they return to me for conventional treatment. They never agree to my requests to go back online to point out the pitfalls so that fellow sufferers are not similarly deceived. I'm not sure it would matter if they did. One man I advised against travelling pulled out his wallet, took out a photograph of his four young children and said, 'Look, Doctor – I have to do anything I can to be there for them, regardless of scientific proof.'

What can you say to that? An MS diagnosis from a neurologist leaves so many questions unanswered, it's understandable that people want to try whatever is out there.

I have sent the occasional person to reputable UK clinics for this procedure. These were cases where we had tried and failed with every other treatment option and where the MS was still very active despite all of our attempts at therapy. Sadly, so far it has not been effective for any of my patients. In the right hands, with patients that get treatment at the optimal time, it can be successful, so the future of transplants looks much brighter than even a few years ago.

I guess cognitive biases push us to google what we want to read and I tell patients that I do not blame them in the slightest. I even wonder whether I will follow suit when my own neurological diagnosis is made. After all, I have diagnosed many a doctor with motor neuron disease, MS or Parkinson's and they seek alternative therapies almost as much as non-doctors. I don't blame them either, as hope is an extraordinary thing and I no longer underestimate the power of placebo effects as I once did.

It seems to me that many people's attitude to medication – for MS and other conditions – is formed by their need to be in control. As I mentioned earlier, time and again when I take a history, and ask what medication a patient is on, they don't mention vitamin supplements or complementary therapies. But people spend small fortunes on largely unproven complementary and alternative therapies, and yet baulk at the suggestion that proven medication, which the state will provide practically free of charge, might help them more. So I have concluded that this is about control: medicine is prescribed by a doctor and supported by medical research that can be quite technical and inaccessible, and alternative therapies are self-prescribed by the patient based on their own research, anecdotal and online. And even when someone with MS is doing very well on state-subsidized medication, it is not uncommon for them to attribute their well-being to their regime of reiki and Pilates. Again, whatever works.

On a related note, patients commonly ask, sensibly, what side effects the drugs I might prescribe could have. And I usually explain that the first effect will be, hopefully, to alleviate their MS symptoms, their headaches, their pain or their seizures. Then I'll list the most common reported side effects, thereby risking the 'nocebo' effect, where describing potential side effects leads to a patient being more likely to experience them – and thus being less likely to take the tablets and benefit from their positive effects. It is a difficult line to walk when trying to help someone, while still giving full disclosure and risking scaring off the poor patient altogether.

This preoccupation with side effects applies to all patients equally, most remarkably young people, who will list off all sorts of illicit drugs they've taken over a weekend of partying at a music festival: ketamine, 'a few E', a little cocaine and several buckets of alcohol. They may even realize that this overindulgence has caused the fits that have brought them into Casualty or into my clinic. And yet they ask suspiciously about the potential side effects of the anti-seizure medication I prescribe. At such moments I like to imagine them shouting over the blaring music, interrogating their dealer about side effects as they hand over pills or some other mystery substance.

Abnormal reactions to medication are not uncommon, so we always check if a patient has had any allergies to drugs in the past. One of the most important discoveries in the twentieth century was penicillin, and Alexander Fleming would be turning in his grave to hear people casually respond that they 'might have' had a reaction to penicillin when they were younger. As a result, for the rest of their lives, they will not be given one of the greatest drugs medicine has to offer for fear of causing harm. As drug allergies can make it difficult to find the right medications for patients who need them, I always urge students to probe deeper as to what each allergic reaction was; it may turn out not to be a true allergic reaction – someone simply felt nauseous after taking a particular antibiotic or painkiller. That's a risk we – and likely they – would be willing to take to save their life, or to help treat a serious disease.

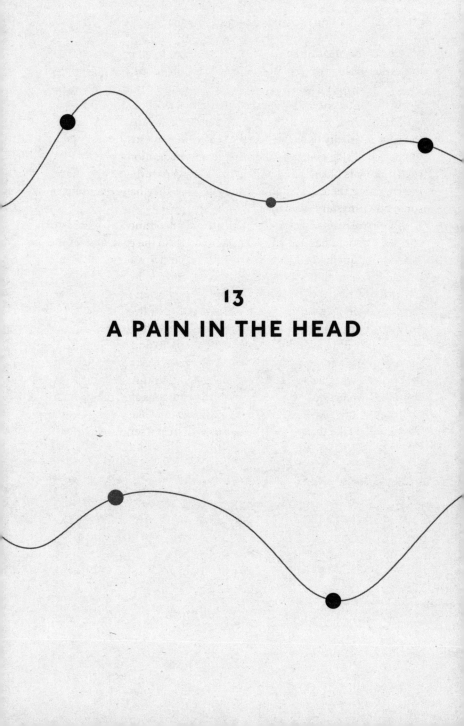

13
A PAIN IN THE HEAD

Mark was forty-five years old and had migraine headaches 'twenty-four/seven' for over twenty years. Your heart sinks as a young doctor when faced with such a story, but the more experienced physician relishes the challenge of such a case. Disregarding the constant pain, he had held down a steady job in finance. His last few years had been very stressful at work and his migraines had escalated in severity and frequency. He had recently separated from his wife and blamed his marital problems on the irritation caused by his constant pain. He blamed the stress at work as the cause of his migraines. He drank to help alleviate the stress. The drinking was negatively affecting his migraines and his marriage, and on it went. The vicious cycle had led to his life falling apart. 'If only I could get the migraines under control, everything would be OK.' His single-mindedness in the face of his illness meant that he was taking no responsibility for the knock-on effects that he had some control over. The idea that the rest of his life would fall back into place once his headaches were cured was fixed in his mind.

He had started taking paracetamol with increasing frequency and moved on to Nurofen and then Solpadeine. By the time I met him he was taking some sort of analgesia three or four times a day.

'Do they help?' I asked.

'No, it's like taking Smarties.'

Mark had sought help from various doctors over the years and, obviously, because he was coming to see me with a twenty-year history of pain in his head, things had not gone well. Mark clearly did not like doctors, but I think at this stage Mark did not like anyone. He was angry and frustrated about his headaches, but this was translating into an anger and frustration at his entire life. While he continued to take the over-the-counter painkillers, he also had resorted in recent years to the internet.

I listened to Mark as he showed me page after page of the research papers he felt I should read so I would understand the particular details of his predicament. He had a beautifully organized, colour-coded, Excel spreadsheet for the preceding six months outlining the pattern of his headaches. He had converted his 'data' into both bar graphs and line graphs. 'I could do a scatter plot for you if you would find it easier,' he offered helpfully. He had a low-grade pain all the time ('the blue line, Doctor') but superimposed on his pain were disabling pains ('the red line') that took him out of action for days on end. He was going to lose his job, his wife, his children – he was at rock bottom.

He spoke quickly and appeared, initially, to have no interest in what I might have to say. When he had finished speaking he exhaled heavily, looked at me with a challenging stare and said, 'That is my story, what can you do for me?' He held my gaze for longer than was comfortable and, if I am honest, I felt a little threatened.

I looked over his spreadsheet and complimented him on his thoroughness. 'I'm a financial analyst – this is what I do,' he said. It is so interesting to see people like Mark drawing on their area of expertise to try and regain control over their medical problems. A librarian, for example, will similarly have organized charts detailing the arc of their symptoms. A doctor, on the other hand, may be the least pragmatic about their symptoms, and jump to their own diagnosis. It is then my job to try to confirm or refute their conclusions.

Neurologists are pretty good at treating migraines with medications both for the acute attacks and to prevent attacks when they are frequent and severe. But it is not as simple as that. Mark is a good example of the multifaceted approach one must take with any patient when looking at the physical, psychological and social ramifications of their illness. Even the most amateur anthropologist could see how muddy the waters of Mark's problems had become. If someone is taking over-the-counter painkillers on more than fifteen days each month, they will get 'medication overuse' headache. In other words, the so-called cure is at least part of the overall disease. The Solpadeine takes the edge off the pain temporarily but, as the effects wear off, the person gets a rebound headache that will prompt a need for more pain relief. Over time they become gradually physically and psychologically dependent on these tablets. With the dependence on medication people will become anxious and their sleep patterns more erratic. Now tired and despondent, some, like Mark, start to drink to help them sleep. Plainly, too much alcohol leads to more headaches. So poor Mark had a combination of migraines, hangovers, medication overuse headaches and sleeplessness. And that is before you consider day-to-day migraine inducers like the pressure of work and the trials of life in general. Mark's life was falling apart over what his friends and family could only see as his 'bad headaches'. And as their reserves of sympathy ran out, Mark became isolated, depressed and ultimately very bitter.

I explained that I felt I could indeed help him, but that he now had four or five problems beyond his migraine and we would have to break each one down and tackle it separately. The easiest one was that he was taking too many 'Smarties'. When he admitted that they weren't working anyway, I asked why he bothered taking them.

'If I don't, I'll be in agony,' he said, so it seemed they were helping some of the time.

Mark saw the logic in what I was proposing and his attitude changed quickly. We agreed he would start by weaning himself off the Solpadeine and other painkillers over the coming month.

We skirted around the question of alcohol. 'I don't drink that much – a few glasses of wine with dinner and pints at the weekend,' he said. And then, to his own surprise, he added, 'That's too much, isn't it?' I suggested he try to cut back.

We discussed ways to try to improve his sleepless nights without alcohol and I gave him broad guidelines for sleeping better (e.g. taking a gentle walk after dinner; cutting back on caffeine; making a list before retiring to try to minimize the raging thoughts that wake us all in the middle of the night; keeping screens – phone or TV – out of the bedroom).

'There are other things we can do,' I said. 'You grind your teeth and clench your jaw when stressed, and we can see from the examination that this has caused laxity of the joints around your jaw. Now you will have more pain in your jaw joints contributing further to head and face pain.'

'Oh, my dentist spotted that and gave me a splint [like a gum shield] to wear at night years ago.'

'But do you actually wear it?'

'No, my wife felt it was, shall we say, offputting.' He smiled at last.

We agreed he would give it another go, and ticked another potentially fixable cause of his chronic head pains off the list.

We were making progress. This is more than half the battle in my view – gaining the patient's confidence and restoring hope that they don't have to serve a life sentence of pain. It was not going to happen quickly I warned, as, after all, he had had headaches for over twenty years. Rather than an immediate cure, we could realistically aim to improve things by 50 per cent over the coming months.

'Months!' he said. 'I don't have months – my wife threatened to divorce me if I didn't keep this appointment today!' (He genuinely had given up on doctors, and had planned on not showing up for the appointment with me.)

On we went down the list. Next, I would arrange some physiotherapy for the tensed muscles of his neck. Finally, I asked him to continue his record-keeping, albeit a tad less obsessively. 'Only fill it in once a day, just before going to bed. Identify the different types of headaches you have had, and see where we are making progress, and where we can do better. Make it more Roald Dahl and less Dostoyevsky,' I said. Finally, he laughed.

I recommended some anti-migraine tablets that he hadn't tried before as a preventative. He was now buoyant, bordering on elated. Having a plan was everything. The man liked a well-conceived plan, after all. It is crucial for people with chronic pain such as Mark's to give not just hope, but a sense that they have regained control of their lives. Mark was determined to try anything, but in my experience this uncomplicated approach works for the majority of people with chronic headaches.

Mark returned a few months later a different person. He was smiling and shook my hand vigorously. He looked healthier and explained that he had followed the plan to the letter. He had a pedometer on his belt and when I asked him about it he said he had been recording over 15,000 steps a day. He still had some headaches, but no longer felt that they were the end of the world. The physiotherapist was marvellous, he said, and she released all of the tension in his neck.

As happens with many middle-aged men, he had gone to extremes. In my experience it is a typical man thing to try to reassert their alpha male status, at least in their own minds. They will listen to doctors but only to a point as many do not like being told what to do – especially by a man of their own age. Whatever advice I might give, the middle-aged man will 'double the dose'. If I suggest they go for an evening walk instead of watching television, they will go out and buy some Lycra and start running as if they were teenagers again. If I suggest a low dose of vitamin D, for example, for people with MS, the middle-aged man will take three or four times the dose suggested.

Mark joined a gym and had taken up running every night; he had given up dairy again (I had not advised this . . .) and was studying mindfulness (. . . nor this); he had worn the dentist's splint and cut out all the non-prescribed drugs he had been taking for years.

In addition, he admitted shamefacedly that having read the instructions on the medication I had prescribed he had decided to try to do without it – another typical bid to reassert control. I rarely push it if people like Mark don't want to take medication for migraines – if the pain is bad enough, I reason, then they can come back to my 'potions' if they need to.

'I still have headaches about once a week, but I can see the progress I have made and aim to take on the second half of the pain over the next three months,' he said. Now, with half his pain eliminated, three months didn't seem such a long time to hope for a resolution. I knew he would not be fully cured, but now he had the tools to manage the chronic headaches, and more importantly he had regained control of his life.

Not everyone with chronic headaches embraces the treatment regime that Mark did. Many fall back into old habits after some small initial victories. Some people with chronic headaches give up on conventional medicine. Such is their desperation that they will take advice from anywhere – online, friends, colleagues, fellow pub-goers – on the scantiest of evidence. Usually, they give up dairy first. Then they will take on all sorts of other dietary restrictions. This is often followed by supplementing with St John's Wort and Butterbur, for which there is a little evidence of effectiveness for some people, though it's not very scientific. They wear copper bracelets to 'ward off' headaches. Inevitably they will try acupuncture and variations of reflexology. I've heard an increasing amount about cranio-sacral therapy of late. And yet, here they are, sitting in front of me looking for a cure. But you cannot fix everything that contributes to the problem, and nor is it a doctor's job to do so – Mark's marriage never recovered, for example – but you can at least point them in the right direction.

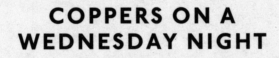

14
COPPERS ON A
WEDNESDAY NIGHT

Most of us get band-like pressure across our foreheads from time to time when our work or home lives become overwhelming. We take a couple of paracetamol and get on with our lives. For a significant proportion of people, however, headaches can be much more severe and sometimes totally incapacitating.

Pain in the head is different from, say, a pain in the knee or the shoulder, for the simple reason that we cannot examine our own heads very well; we cannot see or massage the injured area satisfactorily. Beyond this, the brain within is what makes us who we are, what makes us human. As central as it is to our own identity, the brain is in many ways the great unknown, and thus people's fear may be that pain is the beginning of a fatal illness.

There is astounding variability in how each person suffers with headaches. Some people get fairly mild, infrequent migraines, whereas other people's lives can be ruined by recurrent headaches. Classically someone might get a visual disturbance called an aura and see twinkling lights around their field of vision. This can be followed by difficulties finding the words they want to say; weakness or tingling in their arms and legs; mild confusion; some even appearing detached from their surroundings. The majority end up with a severe throbbing pain on one side of their head. They become sensitive to light and intolerant of noise and have to retire to a dark room and try to switch off from the world while they suffer in silence. I have seen many people in Casualty with such severe headaches that we suspected (as did they) that they might have had a stroke, but the scans were almost always clear.

Migraine affects at least 10–15 per cent of people, often starting in the teenage years, but it can come on at any time. Regularly a patient with migraine will have a family history of migraines, so that tends to make diagnosis a little easier. But for others getting a diagnosis can be tricky. Migraines might start with pains in the stomach, and some people will spend years seeing the wrong doctors. Or they may only get visual blurring with no actual headache, and so think they are going blind.

People with migraine, like with many pain syndromes, do not always get the sympathy they deserve. We cannot see or feel their pain, so 'migraineurs' can feel dismissed by friends and family as being feeble souls. It is very hard to explain just how disabling the headaches are, not to mention the accompanying nausea, vomiting, visual problems and the need to withdraw from the world temporarily. Patients miss work as a result and colleagues tire of having to cover for them, further undermining their self-esteem.

When I started in neurology I found my limited ability to deal with patients' chronic headaches extremely frustrating, and what progress we made rather unrewarding. I think that is because, when you start out studying neurology as a young doctor, you focus on the more 'exciting' areas – movement disorders like Parkinson's or conditions like MS – where there is a lot of novel research activity and the stakes for both patient and doctor are very high. Over 90 per cent of the headaches I diagnose are migraine, tension or medication overuse headaches, or a combination thereof, and you soon realize that, thankfully, the vast majority of the people you will see with headaches do not have a life-threatening problem.

Because headaches are so common your great fear as a doctor is that you will miss one of the potentially lethal causes of some headaches. We have been accused by media commentators and bloggers of over-investigating people with headaches, and this is probably true, but missing a diagnosis of a brain tumour or haemorrhage doesn't bear thinking about, either for the patient or for the doctor.

Anne was in her second year in physiotherapy in college when she made an appointment to see me. She had a dry wit and she wasn't in the least fazed by the whole 'medical palaver' as she called it. She had moved to Dublin a few years previously and was sharing a flat with three other young women. She described her lifestyle in hilarious detail.

She would go out at least three nights a week. These evenings would start with some 'prinks' (she really was getting into the Dublin lingo), consisting of either wine or gin, as Anne and her friends got ready for the night ahead. They would then go out and consume many pints, followed by shots while out clubbing until the early hours. Once in a while she would take half an ecstasy tablet – 'Only if I was exhausted,' she added, by way of mitigation. She would get home around two or three in the morning, and was up for college at 9 a.m.

Her diet had gone 'pear-shaped', she said, 'much like myself'. She and her flatmates ordered home delivery four or five nights a week. Anne was about five foot four in height and weighed fourteen stone – she had put on three stone since starting college. Her skin had become 'teenage' once more, so she had been started on minocycline, an antibiotic for acne, by her GP. She was on the pill and blamed this for the weight gain, but admitted her lifestyle was probably not helping.

Anne flicked through her iPhone to show me pictures taken on her school graduation day a couple of years earlier. Though she introduced the subject, I did not comment on her weight gain. It is a minefield for a doctor when an overweight patient is in front of you. You do not want to offend them, particularly if they are already self-conscious about their size, and we have all heard horror stories of doctors jumping in with both feet and blaming all a person's problems on their weight. Apart from being a foolish thing to do before examining a patient thoroughly, it's not helpful to patients who are very likely to know themselves that they are carrying some excess weight. After all, Irish families don't tend to hold back in telling loved ones – 'for their own good' – that they're getting a bit heavy. So I usually ask even the biggest patients I see whether they have lost or gained any weight in the months prior to seeing me. It is lovely to see an overweight person beam with pride at this question and tell me how they have lost a few pounds. At least you know that they recognize that their weight might be a health issue and are doing something to help themselves, so it is a great starting point for helping them yourself.

Anne had started a new diet every month for the last four months, so again regaled me with bittersweet stories about her various attempts to lose weight. 'I gave up carbs in January – I lasted two weeks. I went gluten-free, and that was easier as even Deliveroo cater for that now, but I could not resist the Sunday morning fry-ups.' Then she listed a dizzying range of diets, many new to me – the caveman diet; the 5:2; Atkin's (I had heard of that one) – all of which had ended in failure – 'mostly by Wednesday evening', she said ruefully.

At weekends she returned home to Athlone to recover from college life, bringing along a bag of laundry that her mother would have washed and ironed for her 'little girl' before she caught the Sunday afternoon bus back to Dublin.

'I feel like I have two lives. At home I will go into my old routine of good food and lots of sleep, only to prepare myself for all the late nights back up in Dublin. It's brilliant craic!'

It was when she started to notice she was hard put to read the slides during lectures that she wondered if she might have a problem. She got new glasses, which helped for a while, but she felt that the glasses then started to cause mild headaches, so she had the prescription changed. Over the next few weeks, the headaches worsened and her blurred vision became more persistent. She had started to hear strange sounds, like a tap left running; 'My friends think I am going mad, as I keep checking the sink.' She realized she could not put her symptoms down to her near-constant hangover any longer.

I examined her and gave her an eye test. Even with her glasses on she missed the lower lines on the chart entirely. I looked at the back of her eyes with an ophthalmoscope, which we use to examine the retinae. On each retina, the optic discs look like little saucers at the back of our eyes. With magnification, you should be able to see lots of blood vessels, like strands of spaghetti falling into the plughole of the kitchen sink. If you isolate one strand and follow it along its course, you will eventually see it disappearing down the edge of the plughole – this is the optic disc. The margins of this disc should be well defined. In Anne's case the margins were blurred and looked swollen. The pressure in the fluid in her brain was gradually building, and this pressure had spread to the eye (optic) nerves, causing the optic discs to swell.

This pressure on the optic nerves is what was causing her blurred vision. This is called papilloedema, and is often a harbinger of serious underlying problems in the brain. Most worryingly, it can be a sign of a brain tumour; I have seen people go to their local Specsavers for a routine eye exam, only to have such papilloedema discovered. The next thing they know, they're in Casualty waiting for their fate to be decided by a brain scan. It is very frightening for them, but thankfully the worst-case scenario does not always apply.

Anne's weight gain, the pill, the antibiotic – all three were potentially contributing to the increased pressure in her head and causing her vision and hearing problems. If we did nothing, the pressure would continue to rise and she might go blind. It is an odd feeling sitting in front of someone as they nonchalantly crack jokes and tell tales of wild nights out while knowing that the true situation is so serious. I said only that we needed to act swiftly and organized a brain scan for later that day.

Some people with this condition – originally called 'benign' intracranial hypertension, until we realized that the 'benign' element was not always the case – have an underlying clot in the veins draining the blood back from their brain to their heart, and the 'blocked drain' leads to the raised pressure. Anne's brain scan revealed no such clot, so we proceeded to a spinal tap, or lumbar puncture.

Almost everyone I meet shudders when I mention that we will be doing a lumbar puncture. It involves lying on your side and curling into a foetal position with your back to the doctor, who cleans the area around the lower back with iodine or alcohol swabs and gives a local anaesthetic injection, like the one you get when you are having dental work. Then we place a long skinny needle into the numbed area. The patient feels pressure as we push the needle gently towards the outside part of the spinal cord.

The purpose is to get a sample of the fluid that surrounds the spinal cord, called the cerebrospinal fluid (CSF). The spinal cord and brain are bathed in this liquid, and so it is like testing the water in which our brains and nerves are 'swimming'. Think of it as like testing the level of chlorine in a swimming pool.

It is an extremely informative test as it allows us to measure the finely tuned pressure of the fluid around the brain and spinal cord. It also allows us to test the content of the fluid and we use it to check for meningitis, bleeding in the brain and MS, among other things.

The lumbar puncture is done for many reasons, depending on the hospital department and why the patient is there. For instance, in Casualty it is often done for suspected meningitis (inflammation and infection of the covering of the brain) and encephalitis (inflammation or infection of the brain tissue itself).

The procedure generally lasts about twenty minutes, but can take

longer: arthritis makes it difficult to get in between bones and liga-
ments that are less flexible; some people are heavier than others, and
it can be difficult to get the spinal needle through fatty tissue. When
a patient becomes distressed we will postpone the procedure, and re-
arrange it for another time (if time allows) or organize for the needle to
be placed under the guidance of x-rays. Mostly there are no problems,
but lumbar punctures tend to get a bad reputation online as people
seem to be quick to report a bad experience but don't bother if they
have a good one.

A harder job for the doctor makes it harder still for the patient, especially when they can't see what is being done, or even see the doctor.
Occasionally the needle might touch a nerve, causing a shooting pain
down the leg, which is very frightening and makes patients fear they'll
be paralysed. If I'm honest, I dread the day I'll have one myself, but
there is no getting around how essential they are as a diagnostic tool.

As Anne lay on her side, we gave the local anaesthetic. For the first
time, I saw that she was afraid, and I felt so sorry for her. She was trying to be cool and brave, but suddenly this bright young woman's jocular façade fell away. She started to cry when she recognized that there
might be something seriously wrong. The nurse held her hand as we
put the long needle into the space between the bones near the bottom
of her spine.

It is extremely satisfying when the clear fluid suddenly starts to flow
into the test tubes. With Anne, the spinal fluid shot out, and we attached
a pressure monitor. Normally the pressure gauge would read less than
20 centimetres of water (the fluid flows out and climbs up the vertical
monitor slowly and comes to a rest around the 15–20 mark). Anne's fluid
climbed rapidly beyond the 20 mark, then the 30 and then the 40, eventually spurting out of the top of the monitor and on to the curtains.

It was as high a reading as I had ever seen, and the fluid flowed for
nearly another minute until we could see the pressure start to drop
again slowly. We removed enough fluid to allow the mark to fall back
below the requisite 20 mark and removed the spinal needle. Although
she could not see what was happening she instantly felt better: 'I feel
clearer in my head already, less muzzy.'

I let Anne lie still for an hour and came back to see her. 'My headache is gone!' she exclaimed. 'I can see properly again!' It was remarkable; usually someone does not feel such rapid relief, so I presume there was an element of a placebo effect from the relief of not being diagnosed with a clot or a tumour and realizing that this was all very treatable.

We agreed she would do her bit to help herself and I would do mine. I gave her some medication to help keep the pressure down, but explained that it would be far more effective in the medium term if she lost some weight, gradually, and if she went off both the pill and the antibiotic.

A few months later she returned looking practically radiant. Her complexion was healthier and she had lost a stone in weight. The headaches had gone, and she no longer needed glasses. She was chuffed with herself. I checked in on 'college life'.

'Well, I won't lie to you,' she said. 'I gave my nightclub VIP card to a friend for a while, but life goes on, doesn't it? I have given up Jäger-bombs altogether. I stay in on Mondays and Tuesdays now, but I can't be expected to be a hermit, can I?' She laughed. 'And I've lost weight and tried to improve my diet.'

Anne was back to being the bubbly character I had first met. Soon, I hoped, she would forget the whole experience, for is that not the point of what we are doing? To return the unwell to wellness, both physically and psychologically? I wanted Anne to return to normal – and, apparently, there is no better 'normal' for a country girl in college than Copper Face Jack's of a Wednesday night.

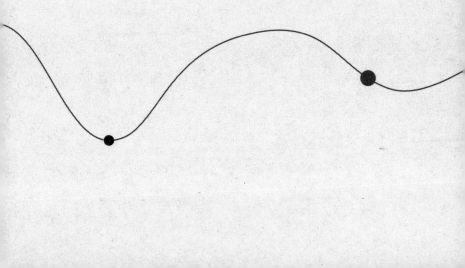

15
LIKE FATHER, LIKE SON

Adam's father had won a Senior Cup rugby medal in the 1970s, was a hero to his friends in the golf club and was respected in the local area. Adam had resolved he would be the same. He started running each evening, mile after mile. Initially he trained with his schoolmates every morning, and then on his own at lunchtime. He felt he needed to bulk up so he started with protein shakes twice a day, and then graduated to all sorts of supplements that the guys at the gym swore by.

The gym membership was a Christmas present from his father. Adam could see how proud his dad was when he went from playing on the third team, to the seconds and was finally on the cusp of a place on the school's first team. He pushed himself harder at every weights session, and was more than satisfied with his progress.

On a wet Thursday evening at his weekly appraisal at the gym he and his coaches decided that he was ready to up the weights he was lifting. After the fourth or fifth attempt to lift the weights above his head, he felt a crack in his neck. He described later how something had gone 'pop' in his brain. He collapsed on the floor and was lucky the weights did not fall on top of him. He lost consciousness briefly. He woke on the ground, with his friends looking down at him. He got up slowly and felt a wave of dizziness, so sat down again quickly. He was embarrassed but insisted he was OK – 'just a bit light-headed'. But something told him that all was not well.

In spite of his worries, he was acutely aware of not showing weakness – one of the players from the Cup team had been prohibited from playing for the rest of the season after being knocked out in a practice session a few weeks earlier. So Adam put on a brave face and told the others that he hadn't eaten earlier – 'probably just low blood sugar', he said. He went for a walk on his own and felt better quickly.

Ignoring the coaches' advice to take it easy for a while, within the hour he started lifting some lighter weights. No problem there, so he pushed on. When he got to the machine where he had collapsed earlier, he was nervous but eased into it. As he relaxed, his competitive instinct kicked in. He was close to the higher weight again when he began to feel it. As he strained, he felt a sharp pain at the top of his head. He panicked, and dropped the weights. He stood up quickly, but collapsed again.

His friends were really concerned now, but he assured them he was fine and that he had just overdone it. He showered and left the gym, hoping against hope that his friends would keep quiet about the episodes. He felt fine by the time he got home, but homework was out of the question as he couldn't concentrate, so he went to bed early. The next morning he woke up feeling fine. He went to the bathroom, and after a few minutes in the shower a niggling pain in the base of his skull made itself felt. It got progressively worse, and by the time he had dressed he had an excruciating headache.

'Oh God,' he thought, 'I've burst a blood vessel in my head. I won't be able to play.' He lay down on his bed and was relieved to feel the headache dissipating. He told himself that he was overreacting and just needed to calm down. When the pain had subsided he decided he had better get going or he would miss pre-school rugby training. He stood up nervously, but he was fine. Yet by the time he was on the bus the pain had started to return. In the changing room his head was pounding and he felt dizzy again. He had to tell someone. His coach asked if he'd been out the night before. When Adam said no, the session was cancelled and his coach drove him to Casualty.

We arranged an MRI scan during which the scanning process was halted briefly and dye was injected into Adam's veins. The beautiful pictures of Adam's brain showed that there was no tumour, no bleeding and no inflammation, but the covering of the brain and spinal cord – the meninges – lit up after the dye was injected.

Adam had a low-pressure headache – the opposite of Anne's high-pressure. When he had strained himself lifting the heavier weights, he had torn a tiny hole in the meninges. The brain is like an orange – the fruit is the brain itself and the meninges is like the peel that forms a protective covering (membrane) around the precious tissue. The cerebrospinal fluid lies between the fruit and the peel and acts to bathe the brain and spinal cord and helps protect against external stresses to our skulls. When we do a lumbar puncture, as with Anne, we sample the fluid between the meninges and the brain/spinal cord. We then take the needle out and leave a tiny hole in the protective covering that seals up quickly in most people. In others, like a stubborn nick of the razor when shaving, the injury refuses to heal and the spinal fluid can continue to leak out. If it does, the patient will get an almighty headache whenever they sit up which is relieved only by lying flat. This can go on for days or even weeks.

This was basically what was happening to Adam; the tiny tear was allowing the cerebrospinal fluid to leak out, like a dripping tap. When he lay flat, the fluid in the system attained a sort of equilibrium, like a builder's level. But when he stood up, gravity made the fluid flow downwards and seep out of the hole. This 'dehydrated' the brain, causing Adam's severe headaches. The meninges lit up after the dye was injected because of the low pressure in the fluid between the meninges and the brain. This confirmed the low pressure in the fluid protecting Adam's brain.

Fixing an unhealed hole after a lumbar puncture, or a tear like Adam's, requires taking some of the patient's own blood and injecting it into the region where the leak is happening. The patient's blood then does what blood will, and clots. The clot serves to cover over the hole or tear, sealing off the leak. This is known as a blood patch. It can all seem like plumbing, and that's basically what it comes down to.

I called the anaesthetist. Anaesthetists are the best doctors for this kind of thing (they perform epidurals for women in labour and blood-patching is a not dissimilar process). She arrived quickly and took a small sample of blood from Adam and then proceeded to re-inject the blood into his lower back area, which has been shown to help heal any leak in the system. It was not pleasant, but Adam bore the pain stoically. I left him to lie on his back for a few hours while I got on with seeing patients on trolleys around him.

When I returned, Adam was sitting up, smiling. 'The pain is gone,' he said. 'Can I go home?'

From our point of view it was a job well done. A quick diagnosis, nothing too serious, and an expertly executed treatment, all within the space of a few hours.

As is often the case, especially with young healthy people like Adam and Anne, after successful treatment patients quickly consign their fears to the far reaches of their memory and want to get back to their lives.

The Senior Cup rugby tournament was starting in a few weeks. Adam was cured – but would you let your son run back on to a rugby pitch after an event like that? I certainly wouldn't, and told him and his father so. They were dismayed.

'Are you sure?' his father asked.

'No, I'm not sure,' was the only honest answer I could give, 'but he is at risk of another tear. I'd recommend that he sit it out this year.'

Adam started to cry and his father looked at me grimly.

'But you cannot say for sure that he will get this again if he plays?' he asked.

I knew where this was going.

'I really think he should not play,' I said. I pointed out that, were it to happen again, he might not be so lucky, and that I had seen people who have had to have multiple blood patches that didn't work this well, so I felt he had been pretty fortunate.

One Sunday afternoon a few weeks later I was watching the schools rugby on TV and saw Adam receiving the ball on the halfway line. He took off, beat his opposite number at a canter and offloaded in a tackle to his teammate, who ran in for a try. I watched Adam jump to his feet and run around with his friends in celebration. So, my advice about the danger of him playing again had not been enough to convince them that he should miss his big chance to emulate his dad's achievements.

I'm always perplexed when a doctor's advice is wilfully ignored. If he had been injured, would Adam and his father have lived with regret for years to come? Or would they blame me for not being more insistent? But if I had been, would they have listened? I followed Adam's team's progress and was relieved when they lost in the semi-final. His dream was over, but at least he was out of harm's way – for the rest of that season at least.

16

HEAL THYSELF

I fractured my collarbone in my last failed attempt to play rugby at school. I was far too skinny compared with the other boys and, although I loved the game, I was no match for their ever-increasing size. I got hand-tripped as I ran with the ball and fell awkwardly on my outstretched hand causing a searing pain in my neck. I had no idea what had happened, but was taken off the pitch and sent home. I was unable to cut my dinner that evening and complained to my father about the pain. He used my scarf to put my arm in a makeshift sling, cut my food into small pieces and gave me a spoon to use with my left hand. And that was it for the next few days.

After much complaining on my part, he eventually acquiesced and took me for an x-ray; it confirmed I had fractured my collarbone. It had already started to heal imperfectly, however, and there was little to be done at that point, leaving me with a disfigured right collarbone ever since.

It is funny how many of my friends whose parents were doctors had similar experiences. In our early days we would laugh at how dismissive our doctor parents were about the childhood ailments or injuries we may have incurred. It was not a lack of empathy, but when you see genuinely sick people every day, sniffles, cuts, bruises and even fractures – even those of your own children – tend to pale into insignificance. And now we are the case-hardened ones, we will dismiss medical complaints in those closest to us either through denial that there could be something seriously wrong or reminding them that we see far worse things on a daily basis. When any of my siblings complains of a pain it has to be pretty persistent and causing real distress before I will try to help them out medically.

My father had his first heart attack when I had just finished my first year at medical school (pre-med as it was then called). I had found the year extremely arduous, especially having spent so much time the previous two years studying to get into medicine, and I was on the cusp of giving up. I just about scraped through my exams. I might easily have dropped out had I been forced to do repeat exams in the autumn – I just could not have faced further hours of isolated study through the summer.

So it was with great relief that I set off with my father and siblings to Connemara. The car packed up – my dad, five children, aged nine to twenty-two, Ruskin, the red setter, and enough food and clothing for a small army (such was the isolation of our destination) – we set off one Saturday morning for our annual two-week holiday in a tiny cottage that my grandfather owned in the back of nowhere. We were halfway through the six-hour journey (slowed to a crawl by the need for regular pit stops for food and toileting and occasionally to clear the car of canine flatulence, or worse) when my father developed pains in his chest. He pulled the car over in a hotel car park in Athlone.

Though supposedly an expert in biology, chemistry and physics, I was of absolutely no use medically or otherwise; I couldn't even drive. He sent the three younger kids for a walk (on their own!) around the town and my older sister and I tried to persuade him to go to the local hospital. He wouldn't hear of it and, after an hour's rest, he lit up a smoke and off we went again.

By Galway the chest pains had recurred and, despite my youth, even I could tell something was seriously wrong and I insisted that he go to Casualty. He had an electrocardiogram (ECG) to assess what was going on with his heart. I had no idea how to read an ECG at that point and didn't know enough to fake asking intelligent questions. In my eyes, the young senior house officer on duty might as well have been the heart transplant pioneer Christiaan Barnard himself – I regarded him as the man who could save the situation. I attempted to talk him into keeping my dad in hospital. My older sister and I told Dad we would sort out accommodation for ourselves and the younger kids. Although he wavered for a few moments, he thought better of it and discharged himself against the advice of his younger colleague. Perhaps it was a typical older doctor's scepticism about the judgement of a novice, or perhaps he was being stoic for the sake of his children.

Whatever it was, he drove on to our grandfather's cottage perched on the edge of the Atlantic – miles from a telephone. The nearest shop or pub was at least a half-hour's walk, and the nearest hospital was the one we left behind in Galway, over an hour's drive away. For the next three days I fretted as my normally active father lay in bed in the back room. Gradually the chest pains subsided. He never complained. He must have been worried beyond belief. We crept around the house as quietly as possible but, given there were six people in three rooms and a dog convinced he could consume the entire local flock of sheep, it was not quite the ideal coronary care unit.

A few days later he was up and about again and, keen to keep the holiday going, started taking us out on the local lake for our customary fishing expeditions. These took place in a leaky boat that had a small pot to bail out the brown water that gathered at our feet. With all six of us piled in, no life jackets and an excitable dog on board too, it was a miracle that any of us survived those health and safety-free summers.

Though he appeared to recover quickly, years later tests would confirm that my father had had a potentially life-threatening cardiac arrest that summer. It haunts me still to think how easily the second Doctor Tubridy could have died in Galway that weekend.

When we got back to Dublin, I tried to persuade him to go to see someone about his heart but I don't know if he did. He was, at that point, rather fatalistic about life as the separation made him a little melancholic for a few years, and he had a lot to deal with at work too.

He never complained once about being unwell. At the time I thought this admirable but in retrospect his inability to accept himself as a patient seems foolish. Indeed, whenever I brought up the events of the summer he would almost get irritated and mutter something about it all being fine and that there was no need to worry. Doctors are said to make the worst patients and he was living proof of this. We ate our usual diet and we both drank to excess at times. He smoked away for many more years and never seemed to have another problem until years later, although it is more likely he just never told me.

After my first year of medical school, I seemed to settle into the routine and the study more. Midway through medical school, doubts about the path I was on resurfaced. I was working as a waiter in Melbourne for the summer and having the time of my life. I was making good money on tips and saving to pay back the loans I had taken to travel abroad. The sense of independence while earning my own money was exhilarating because at home most of each year was spent studying and I was reliant on the generosity of my father for any sort of social life. Having spent three years as a student, I had three more to go. And even after qualifying as a doctor, I would then be going back to the bottom of the medical food chain once again. I would not be progressing with my life, as I saw it, until I was in my late twenties, which seemed so far off when I had just turned twenty-one. I resolved to stop studying medicine and join the real world, hoping to run a restaurant of my own in due course.

Fuelled by too much Australian beer, I called my father in Dublin to tell him of my decision. Far from shouting and screaming down the phone he quietly suggested I come back to Dublin in September and see how I felt after a few more months before changing course. Thank God he did.

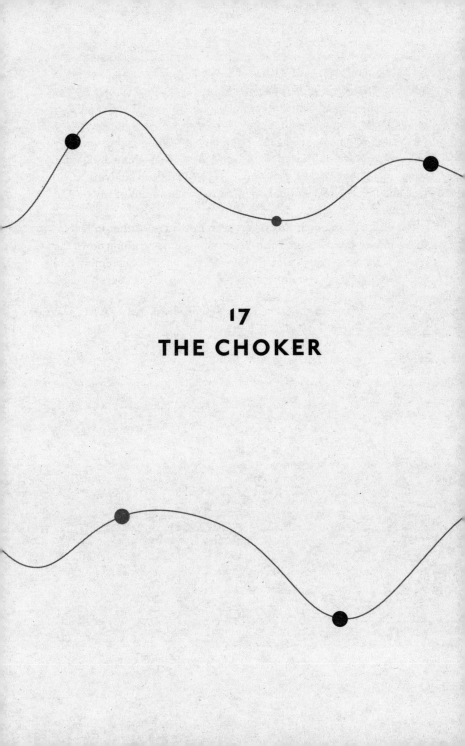

17
THE CHOKER

Joanne was celebrating her fortieth wedding anniversary with her husband, Neil, in a posh restaurant just off the Boulevard Saint-Germain when the third piece of her bœuf bourguignon got stuck in her throat. She coughed, and reached for her water glass, but very quickly a wave of panic hit her as she struggled to catch her breath. Her usually attentive husband seemed distracted by the waiters in their white shirts and black aprons busily ignoring the guests. Joanne felt the blood drain from her face and dropped her glass. She tried to stand, but was now in full fight-or-flight mode and flight was winning.

Neil jumped up in fright, realized what was wrong, but was unsure what to do. He had seen this in movies and in countless medical dramas and, he would tell me afterwards, had even seen someone have their throat cut to relieve a blocked airway. He didn't fancy doing that, so he stood behind her as he had seen Dr House do once on the television, and tried to perform what he called 'the Heimfeld test'. The other diners rushed over to help as he clearly had no idea what he was doing – 'it's not like it is on television when you're trying to save your wife's life' – and pandemonium ensued.

Finally, the waiter casually took over, grabbing her firmly from behind and briskly jerking her body upwards two or three times, whereupon the offensive piece of bœuf flew out of her mouth and on to the floor. Joanne gasped in relief and sat down quickly, embarrassed at the scene she had caused. 'It's OK,' she said to the waiter in a bad French accent, 'the food just went down the wrong way.' She drank some water from Neil's glass, composed herself and tentatively went back to her meal. The waiter was insisting on calling an ambulance, but she brushed him off, too mortified to consider it. He shrugged as only a French waiter can, and left them alone until dessert. Joanne finished her meal slowly, carefully cutting her food into child-sized bites, but was keen to finish so that they could leave.

Over the next few days, they walked many miles around Paris. She was exhausted each evening, but put it down to too much shopping and too much wine. Still, she had a niggling feeling something was wrong. Back in Dublin, all the following week she was drained by eight o'clock each evening and, although she did not choke again, she felt as if there was something stuck in her throat whenever she tried to eat. She put it down to anxiety after the episode in Paris.

A few days later Joanne Skyped her daughter, Alison, a trainee nephrologist, in Sydney. Alison laughed at her story of 'the Heimfeld test' and her mother's humiliation in front of the cool Parisians. She said, 'I can see you've not stopped celebrating yet.'

'What do you mean?' Joanne asked, mildly offended.

'You've hit the wine early this evening!' Alison said with a smile.

'I'll have you know I have not had a drink since we got back.'

'But you're slurring your words,' Alison said innocently.

'No, I am not!' Joanne replied, enunciating in an exaggerated manner – and with some effort, she quickly realized.

'OK, Mum, whatever,' Alison said, and they moved on to other events.

Their Skype calls always upset Joanne. She missed Alison terribly, and regularly ranted at Neil as to why they had brought up their children, and worked hard to educate them, and now Alison was living on the other side of the world. Joanne had come to expect feeling sad as they said goodbye, but felt a shiver of worry when Alison signed off with, 'You know I love you, Mum.' Alison wasn't given to professions of love, and Joanne could see the concern in her daughter's face.

Later that evening, she was chatting to Neil about the call. Unprompted, he asked, 'Well, can I have some of that wine, or did you finish the bottle on your own?'

Furious at this second accusation of solitary drinking, Joanne said, 'What do you mean? I haven't had a drink since Paris. Do I seem drunk?'

'A little,' he replied. 'Your voice sounds a bit slurred, but maybe you're just tired.'

The next morning, after a sleepless night, Joanne found herself looking in the bathroom mirror and attempting to recite the alphabet in as distinct and articulate a way as she could. When she got to 'S', she started to slur.

'I do sound drunk!' she thought. 'Oh my God, I'm having a stroke.' She called Neil and asked him to drive her to Casualty. That's where I saw her a few hours later.

Her CT brain scan was thankfully clear, so there was no evidence of stroke, but her slurred speech was becoming more persistent. She looked forlorn on the uncomfortable trolley, and when she tried to put on a brave face she seemed as expressionless as someone with Parkinson's (in that condition the facial muscles can appear unmoving). I listened to her story and it turned out I had known her daughter when she was one of our medical students.

'Do you want me to call her?' I asked. 'She might be able to help as she was the one to point out there was something wrong.'

Alison laughed when I asked whether she remembered me. 'Jesus, Prof, how could I ever forget? You are one of the main reasons I did nephrology and not neurology!'

I was rueful but you can't win them all; I made a mental note to be nicer in lectures and tutorials in future. I asked Alison what she'd thought after the Skype call with her mum the previous evening.

'I remember a lady in clinic with you who spoke like Mum spoke last night. She had myasthenia gravis and it was the only case of myasthenia I saw when I worked with the neurology team. It stayed with me, though, as she made a great recovery, having sounded like a wino when she came in.'

Alison certainly didn't hold back – her Australian adventure had given her a new confidence since her student days, and I couldn't have been happier for her. In addition, I agreed with her diagnosis, the only time I have seen such brilliant long-distance clinical acumen.

Joanne indeed had a condition called myasthenia gravis (MG) that explained her difficulty articulating words and problems swallowing. There are many different kinds of autoimmune disorders in neurology. MG is a chronic autoimmune neuromuscular disease that causes weakness in the muscles which are responsible for breathing and moving most parts of the body, including the eyelids, arms and legs.

How I explain it to patients is like this: your nerves come from your brain like electric cables, and when your brain sends a signal to the muscles, electricity passes along the cables. When that signal gets to the end of the cable (nerve), there is a small gap for the signal to travel to arrive at the muscle (the neuromuscular junction). Think of it like a postman travelling from the post office with a letter – in this case a letter instructing a muscle to move – and getting as far as the letter box. Usually the postman puts the letter through the letter box and completes a successful delivery. But in MG it's as if the letter box has been sealed off so the letter doesn't get delivered – the muscles don't get the instruction.

When we get a cold or flu, our bodies set up an immune response. In other words, our bodies produce an army of 'good guys', or antibodies, to take out the 'bad guys', or viral infections. This works well most of the time, but sometimes the good guys get over-zealous and start attacking normal parts of the body. The antibodies go rogue and become bad guys themselves. This is described as an autoimmune condition, so your own immune system is attacking you.

To deal with the condition initially we might have to send in synthetic antibodies to neutralize the rogue antibody that's causing the problem. This is called immunoglobulin, and means having a drip in your arm for a few days. Alternatively, we can try to suppress the bad antibodies and their rebellious nature with other medication called steroids.

I went back to Joanne and Neil and explained what Alison and I had discussed. They were even more impressed with their daughter than I was. They joked that they would sue their doctor daughter for missing the diagnosis (I shuddered internally; doctors are not fond of jokes about lawyers being called). I outlined the plan for tests and treatment, and we admitted her to hospital for five days of treatment with immunoglobulin.

Joanne responded well to the treatment and I joined in her next Skype conversation to Alison while she was still on the ward.

'Prof, I'm really sorry if I offended you with my neurology comments a few days ago. I guess you caught me at a bad time,' she said. Confidence regained, but manners never lost.

'You must be tired of Australia by now,' I said. 'Come and apply for some jobs back home.'

Her mum couldn't hide her joy, and shed a tear when Alison said, 'Actually, I was thinking along those lines already, so hopefully . . .'

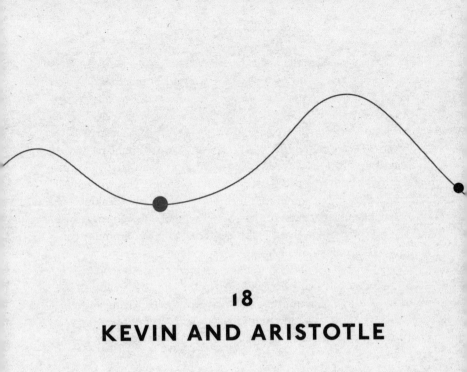

18

KEVIN AND ARISTOTLE

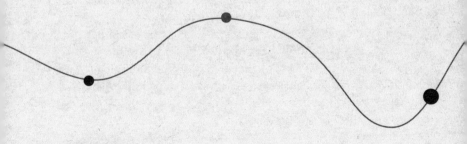

'My wife thinks I look like that sad dog from the *Tom and Jerry* cartoons the kids used to watch on Saturday mornings when they were small. You know the one – sad face, droopy eyes . . . with a monotone voice that always sounds like he's depressed?' Kevin explained. His wife was laughing along with him.

'It's true,' she said. 'We had to look him up but we both remarked how he was starting to look all jowly, like Alfred Hitchcock, and then we remembered the dog in the cartoon. His name was Droopy and he was always deadpan and looked half asleep. That's Kevin for the last six months.'

Kevin was only forty-six years old. He spoke quickly and it was hard to decipher exactly what he was saying. He spoke as if he had cotton balls in his mouth, like Marlon Brando in *The Godfather*. His right eyelid was lying a tad lower than his left, but it was pretty subtle. He saw me watching this and said, 'You think this is bad. It's only early in the morning. Wait until this evening – I'll look like I haven't slept for days. I don't feel tired, and work away as usual but, come seven o'clock, I can hardly keep my eyes open. It varies from day to day, and is much better in the morning, but recently I found myself having to repeat everything when talking at work and the straw that broke the camel's back was when I started to choke on the steak and chips when I was out one night.'

He appeared well, if a little forlorn-looking, but his voice sounded slurred – as if he had had a few drinks that morning. He assured me he hadn't before I even had a chance to ask. Clearly this was an accusation that had been levelled at him before.

I held a pencil up and asked him to follow it with his eyes while keeping his head still. There was no movement and I thought he was not getting it and repeated the instructions a few times. 'I am,' he said, with an air of exasperation. His eyes hardly moved at all.

I held the pen up towards the ceiling and asked him to hold his eyes up 'towards heaven'. He tried his best and, after a minute or so, the right eyelid started to fall slowly, like a window blind being lowered. The left eyelid soon followed suit such that, within another minute, both of Kevin's eyes were practically fully shut.

I examined his arms and legs: they were fine, reflexes responding well and good strength throughout. I gave him a glass of water and asked him to hold some in his mouth for a moment before swallowing so I could stand back and see the effect. Then I instructed him to swallow it back and as he did so the clear fluid came spurting out of his mouth as he coughed it back up and his eyes reddened. 'Shorry about that,' he slurred. Although his wife laughed at the mess, I could see she was worried. I explained that I was pretty sure what it was and that I should be able to confirm it with a few tests.

I got a large cube of ice from the hospital canteen and made him look up once more. As soon as his eyelids tired and the eyelids dropped, I placed the ice cube over the right eye and asked him to hold it there for a minute. We waited. He did not complain about the cold torture I was inflicting upon him. When we took the ice away, the eyelid was almost completely open again.

'That's amazing,' he said. 'But does that mean I will only see properly if I keep my eyes on ice in the future?'

It is touching to see people bear so much, as Kevin had for the preceding weeks and even months, and be so fearful, and still be able to make jokes. I ordered some blood tests and said I'd organize a scan and some electrical tests, but reassured him that what I thought he had was treatable and he exhaled with relief.

'So, it's not motor neuron or MS?'

'No, I think you have a fairly rare condition in which the wires to the eyes are OK. The muscles of the eyes are OK. The problem is the connection between the wires and the muscles, called the neuromuscular junction.'

He looked at me quizzically and I gave him my 'postman' explanation. In Kevin's case I believed that myasthenia gravis explained his droopy eyes, difficulty articulating his words and problems swallowing. Aristotle Onassis, Jackie Kennedy's second husband, could be seen with similar droopy eyes in certain photographs. It is believed that the condition eventually affected his breathing, complications from which ultimately killed him.

'I wouldn't mind his money but he can keep his illness,' Kevin said wryly.

The electrical test I arranged is called an electromyogram, in which a fine needle is put into the affected muscles and the signals are recorded to see how strong they are. When Kevin's muscles were stimulated, for a while they worked well enough, but then the signals became weaker. It all served to confirm the diagnosis.

Kevin's slurred speech and difficulty swallowing certainly could indeed suggest MND. He was overjoyed to know that his condition was definitely myasthenia – his worst fear had been that he would end up 'like that Stephen Hawking guy'. Some years ago, the popular Irish sports commentator Colm Murray went public with his diagnosis of motor neuron disease. He used his media profile to increase awareness of the condition and raise money for various research attempts to understand it. His interviews as his condition deteriorated exposed many Irish people to motor neuron disease for the first time and had a huge impact. Since then it has become customary for his name to come up in consultations with men of a similar age to Kevin – that and a fear of what a few of them call 'super MS'.

It is striking how inattentive we can be when listening to the plight of others. People knew Colm Murray had a very serious neurological disease, but perhaps many did not register that this was motor neuron disease and not MS (hence the 'super MS') – or maybe they thought they were one and the same condition.

Thankfully, Kevin's version of MG was relatively mild and easy to treat. I gave him the 'good guy' antibodies for five days, and then a low dose of steroids and some tablets to keep the postmen from being intercepted en route to his eye muscles. He responded excellently to the treatment and was more than happy to put up with the chore of daily medication to avoid accusations of early-morning drinking. The nickname Droopy soon became redundant.

In spite of having the same label, people with myasthenia can experience its onset in very different ways. And when it comes to treatment, some people need just a few tablets, others an intravenous drip, and some need full-on immunosuppressive drugs with all the dangers that come with a compromised immune system such as infections and even some forms of cancer.

JUST ONE MORE QUESTION

Usually, given a label like myasthenia, patients google it. Luckily in Joanne's case she had her daughter to advise her, because an online search would have revealed the potential devastation the condition can bring. I have seen people become dependent on ventilators for weeks on end, so severe is their form of the disease, and others unable to move their arms or legs or even lift up their drooping heads. It's not a low-risk condition and I'm always mindful of how badly it can turn out.

The variability in reaction to the symptoms is fascinating too. Joanne's feeling of panic when she felt accused of drinking too much wine is in sharp contrast to another MG patient I met around the same time who treated the whole thing as no more than an inconvenience (the lack of broadband in his area may have been a blessing – he too avoided terrifying himself on Google). Frank's myasthenia started when he was driving back to Mayo on the dual carriageway, having come up to Croke Park that morning.

'It had been a long day,' he said, 'and, of course, we lost. But maybe next year . . .'

He had been up at the crack of dawn that morning, and driven three hours to get there. He didn't have a drink, but, ever emotional about his adored Mayo, he had roared his head off throughout their near-annual defeat at the latter stages of the Championship. Deflated but accepting, he set off home with his friends around six o'clock that evening.

'It took nearly an hour to get out of Dublin – how do you ever live in this kip? Anyway, we were trying to make up for the lost time when, around Kinnegad, the lines in the road started to blur. I blinked, and said nothing. Gradually the single lines became double. I thought I was losing it altogether. I drove on, but now there were twice as many cars in each lane in front of me, so I hardly knew where I was.'

'My God, that was very dangerous,' I said. 'I presume you told your friends and pulled the car over?'

'Ah, Doctor, didn't we have to be back for the highlights on the telly? I closed one eye, and everything was grand. So I drove the whole way a bit more slowly with one eye closed – not a bother. It went on like that for a few days and I presumed I was just knackered tired. When I saw the number of cows on the farm had doubled, I decided I was either rich or sick, but that I had better ask Gerry [his GP] to have a look.'

I had a letter from Gerry, who called it straight away: he reckoned that Frank had a sixth-nerve palsy. I mentioned earlier that we have twelve cranial nerves on each side of our heads. These nerves come from the brain and control how we see, hear, eat and smell, among other things. Nerve one controls our sense of smell; nerve two allows us to see the world. Nerve five mediates movement of our muscles of mastication and the sensations we feel on our face. Nerves three, four and six control how we move our eyes. Frank's sixth nerve on the right appeared to be affected, so when he looked to the left, it was OK, but when he looked to the right, the nerve, or the muscle it supplied, failed to work normally and so, instead of one image landing on his retinae, there were two. If he closed his right eye, he 'took out' the damaged part of this exquisitely neat system, and two became one once more.

By the time I saw Frank in clinic a few weeks later, he still had double vision. His MRI scans and blood tests were all clear, so though Frank was none the wiser, his doctor and friend Gerry was much relieved to get confirmation that his instinct was right and that his friend hadn't had a stroke, and didn't have a tumour.

The key to the puzzle was the variation in the degree of his double vision.

'I'm grand in the morning; it's only towards evening that it starts again. I thought I just needed glasses, but the woman in Specsavers says I have 20/20 vision,' Frank said.

Eye strain when driving after a long day or a late night can make the road seem blurry and we will blink rapidly to try and make our vision sharper and to keep from nodding off. However, if we have myasthenia, the lines in the road will remain blurred, or even appear in duplicate, until the eyes are rested – and will go double again at the first sign of fatigue. This will continue until the myasthenia is treated. So, as Frank's day went on, the number of 'letters' getting through to keep his eye muscle working was diminishing, and eventually the muscle ground to a halt. Happily he responded excellently to minimal medication and he has been grand ever since.

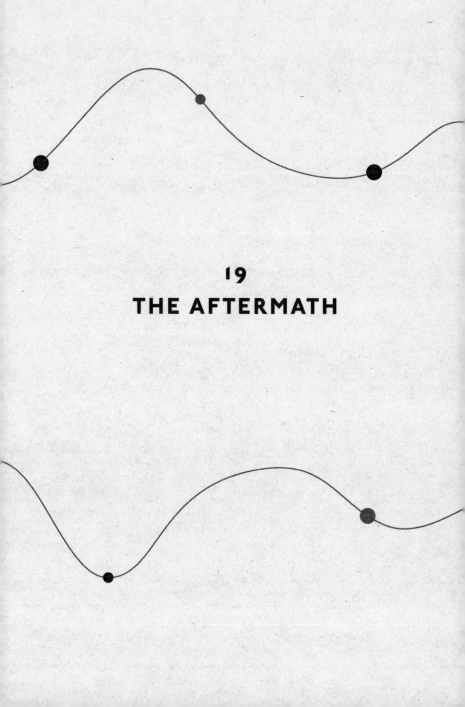

19
THE AFTERMATH

'I was lying on a beach in Marbella and I felt awful,' Susan began. 'We'd been there a week, and I'd developed the most dreadful runs, so I was convinced I'd got food poisoning.' Determined not to ruin the family holiday, Susan tried her best to join in the fun each evening, but then got a pain in her lower back. Susan was only forty-three years old, and was proud of her fitness regimen, but by the third day of the trip she had to abandon her usual morning jog. In between trips to the bathroom she wasn't able to concentrate on her novel, but gamely went to the beach each morning with her husband and two children. Her eldest son had recently turned fifteen and was developing a worrying addiction to his iPhone, and she wanted to keep an eye on him.

She was lying on the sun lounger when she noticed pins and needles in her left foot. She assumed she was just stressed from the persistent diarrhoea and the constant arguing with her son. She jiggled her foot and the sensation abated, but as the afternoon wore on the pins and needles recurred. She only began to panic when her right foot started to develop a similar sensation.

'It was like there was something crawling under my skin. All I could think of were those weird worms you see people in Africa get infected by and burrowing into their eyes.'

She kept her worries to herself and went for a walk, but the back pain was getting worse. When she lay back down she stumbled over the sun lounger, knocking over her husband's cocktail.

'I knew I was in trouble then,' she later recalled. 'I could still feel the creepy-crawlies under my skin, and now I was losing the strength of my legs.'

Her husband helped her to her feet, took her arm and they stumbled awkwardly back to their hotel. 'They must have thought we were both pissed.'

Lying on the bed in her room she started to google her symptoms on her son's confiscated phone, and was relieved when the results suggested that she might have slipped a disc in her back, causing her legs to be weak. 'I kept coming up with sciatica. All the websites said I should just rest so that is what I did.'

She slept fitfully, but the next morning when she reached for the bedside light and realized that her hands were now weak as well she screamed in panic. Her son came in from the adjoining room and she told him to google again while her husband called an ambulance. He found MS and motor neuron disease, but didn't tell her. Eventually, he decided she might have a rare condition: myasthenia.

They went to the hospital and were told she probably had picked up food poisoning all right, and that it was causing a part of her immune system to attack her nerves. They did a scan of her lower back and there was no evidence of a slipped disc. A scan of her brain ruled out MS, the doctors told her.

'Jesus, I hadn't even thought of that,' she said.

Their flights home to Ireland were scheduled for later that evening, and she insisted on travelling, against their advice. She was pushed to the boarding gate in a wheelchair, feeling scared and miserable, and resolved to go straight to hospital in Dublin. That's where I saw her early the next morning.

'Is it myasthenia?' she asked me straight away. 'Will you be able to fix it?'

She couldn't stand without help, and when I asked her to grip my fingers tightly she could barely form fists. Her eyes moved normally, and she was speaking clearly. As I wielded the tendon hammer she was quick to spot I was unable to make her knees 'jump up'.

'That looks bad,' she said, and started to cry.

When I scratched her feet she perked up: 'I can feel that – that's good, isn't it?'

Having tested the motor part of her nervous system, running from the brain to the hands and feet, I moved on to test the wires going in the opposite direction – the sensory nerves. I placed a vibrating tuning fork on the top of her chest and asked could she feel the buzzing sensation.

'Of course I can,' she said, indignantly. The blood drained from her face when I placed the same tuning fork on her big toe, then her ankle and then her knee.

'I can't feel anything. Are you sure it's vibrating?' she cried. 'Am I looking at a wheelchair for ever, Doctor?'

Susan had Guillain-Barré syndrome, a more usable name than its official one: acute inflammatory demyelinating polyneuropathy. She had picked up a bacterium called *Campylobacter jejuni* – a common cause of food poisoning, like salmonella – that had caused her diarrhoea. Her immune system rallied to fight it off, but then had become over-zealous, and started to attack her peripheral nerves (the nerves that also run from the brain but lie outside the brain and spinal cord), gradually stripping them of their insulation (called myelin) that allows speedy conduction of signals to and from the brain. When the sensory peripheral nerves became denuded of their insulation she got the horrible pins and needles. As the attack continued her motor nerves became damaged, causing the weakness and loss of reflexes. The creepy-crawly sensation and the weakness was gradually working its way up her body. Without urgent treatment, it could eventually reach her throat, and affect her breathing and swallowing, and thus could be life-threatening.

Like myasthenia, Guillain-Barré is associated sometimes with a rogue antibody produced by our own defence mechanisms against infections, but where myasthenia attacks the junction between the nerves and the muscles, in Guillain-Barré syndrome the problem is a direct assault on the nerves themselves. So, to return to the postman analogy, whereas in myasthenia the rogue antibody blocks the delivery of a letter just as the postman is trying to put a message through a letter box, in Guillain-Barré syndrome the antibody wrecks the garden path and the postman hasn't got a hope of getting near the letter box to make his delivery.

We performed a lumbar puncture straight away and found that Susan had excessive protein in the fluid surrounding her nerves. This is usually a sign of infection or inflammation in the fluid in which the nerves from the brain are bathed. A further scan with contrast (dye injected into a vein) confirmed the nerve roots were inflamed, causing her low-back discomfort.

We set up the drip for the immunoglobulin and started treatment right away. We also organized electrical tests, but this time for the nerves, not the muscles, and these confirmed our suspicions.

Within a few days Susan was on the mend. Against her better

judgement, she had googled her condition, but stopped reading when she realized how much worse things could have been. Some people respond to treatment quickly, but others can spend months in hospital unable to walk. When I saw a young man with Guillain-Barré syndrome over twenty-five years ago he was staring at a fly that had landed on his left hand. The fly meandered up his forearm and then flitted on to his staring face. I swatted it away gently and he blinked rapidly at me, as if to say 'thank you'. He was conscious; he could hear and see everything – and he could feel the fly on his body, but could do nothing about it. He had developed a rapidly ascending weakness of his legs, arms and facial muscles. He couldn't breathe without the help of a ventilator. His frustration was palpable, and I could only imagine the helplessness he felt. The use of good antibodies for Guillain-Barré syndrome was then in its infancy, so many people who were diagnosed with the condition had to hope that their immune system would stop attacking their nerves, and that the nerves would recover slowly on their own. (That young man was in hospital for many months and eventually transferred to a rehabilitation facility. He survived but required a walking aid for many years and was never able to return to his job as a mechanic. I saw him for a few years for follow-ups, but then he stopped turning up for clinics.)

Susan responded rapidly to the 'good antibodies' and within a week she was walking with a Zimmer frame. 'I thought I wouldn't need one of these until I was eighty,' she smiled ruefully. She recovered slowly over the following few weeks, and when I saw her in the clinic she walked in with a single crutch. Having seen many cases of the same condition with much worse outcomes – including death – I was delighted with her improvement. Her husband, having seen his beloved wife unable to move her arms or legs a few weeks before, was relieved she was alive.

Susan, however, was deeply traumatized by the whole episode. Her time in hospital had taken a serious physical and mental toll. She suddenly looked older than her years. Her recovery was slow but sure; nevertheless her transient dependence on others made her miserable. Her confidence in what she hitherto had taken for granted was shot. She said she felt diminished in front of her friends and family. She felt diminished in front of herself. She was fearful of going outside her own house, such was her loss of self-esteem and confidence. She would not go even as far as the local shops, although physically she appeared able to, as she could not overcome her fear of being seen in public feeling as vulnerable as she was.

It would take many months for Susan to return to some semblance of her former self, but even after a few years she was not the same person psychologically. Eventually I suggested she was recovered and no longer needed her annual check-up visits. I thought she would be cheerful – it is always a good thing, I tell patients, to say goodbye to your neurologist – but she became upset.

'What if it comes back?' she said.

'That's highly unlikely, but I'm here if it does.'

'But would you not just see me, even briefly, once a year – for my peace of mind?'

Naturally, I agreed, and for many years after we met annually and discussed life and the universe – everything except her illness which gradually faded into the annals of her memory.

Often when I try to discharge people from outpatient clinics they will almost plead not to be set adrift. 'Just in case' is their mantra; 'to be on the safe side.' They ask to see me even though the only thing I'm doing is reminding them that they were once ill. They worry that the condition will come back, and need the metaphorical crutch that the doctors who helped them get well will be there if it does. It is sad to see such people – for they are no longer patients in my eyes, even if they remain so in their own – struggle to return to their previous selves.

I meet people many years after I have been involved in their care. Some come running over – always particularly welcome in the neurological world – to celebrate their good fortune with me. But, while many survive neurological illnesses like Guillain-Barré syndrome, some can be left with permanent damage to their arms or legs. I might see such a previous patient in the supermarket, limping away from my oncoming trolley, avoiding saying hello. It is disheartening, but understandable; their successes are my successes, but their sense of failure when their bodies don't fully recover is, in a sense, my failure too.

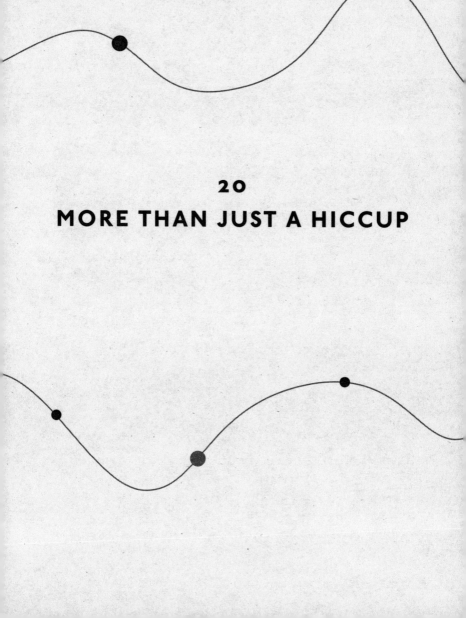

20

MORE THAN JUST A HICCUP

Something as mundane as a hiccup, which we all experience, can be a case of food going down the wrong way or it can herald a cataclysmic brain injury. So while most normal people will wait for an episode of hiccups to blow over, or hold their breath to stop them, a hiccupping neurologist will worry about his brainstem. No wonder we seem weird to many people.

A hiccup is an involuntary spasmodic contraction of the diaphragm followed by the rapid closure of the vocal cords. Hiccup, hiccough or singultus are interchangeable terms used to describe this phenomenon. What causes them and what function they serve in evolutionary terms is not clear. Generally people can get a brief bout of hiccups after consuming particularly spicy food, alcohol or even hot drinks, but they can arise as a result of any condition that irritates the nerves that control the diaphragm (the muscle that controls breathing).

As we all know, hiccups only usually last for a few minutes, or at worst a few hours. Most commonly, they stop suddenly for no obvious reason and some attacks can be stopped by blowing into a paper bag or drinking cold water. Hiccupping that goes on for more than two days is labelled 'persistent', and hiccupping that lasts more than a month is 'chronic'.

The vast majority of cases are benign, but hiccupping can be associated with lung diseases like pneumonia, with kidney failure, and with disorders of the stomach and bowel. Hiccups can also be due to neurological damage in the lowest part of the brainstem, called the medulla. Such conditions include strokes, cancers and infections. So, for example, I have seen people present with hiccupping for days on end as the first sign that they've torn an artery in their neck, which has led to a small stroke.

I was called to Casualty to see Joseph, a 38-year-old Scot who was having difficulty swallowing. Earlier that day he had been doing the front crawl in the swimming pool and after getting out of the water he complained of some pain in his neck. He did not put too much store by it. He had been a rower and had had a fair few neck injuries in his time. But at home an hour or so later he started choking on his evening meal.

He could not swallow the roast potatoes, however small he cut them. Then he started to hiccup, and did not stop.

Joseph's hiccupping was the first sound I heard when I approached his trolley in a pretty chaotic Casualty. He and his wife both looked exhausted and troubled. I explained that I had been asked to have a look to see if there was a neurological cause for his swallowing problems and persistent hiccupping.

His speech was very slurred and I found it hard to understand him, so I proceeded with the examination. The combination of the neck pain, the sudden onset of his symptoms and the slurred speech suggested the hiccups could be due to a vertebral artery dissection – that he had torn a small blood vessel in his neck. He was probably predisposed to a tear like that by his previous injuries and this vulnerability was possibly increased by his vigorous front crawl. As a result of this tear he had had a small stroke in the lower part of his brainstem controlling his swallow and some of his speech mechanisms. The hiccups were also due to this. These certainly seemed to be the most distressing symptom for him.

We arranged an urgent brain scan and identified the damaged blood vessel. The hiccups disappeared after two days and, with the aid of blood thinners to avoid further injury, Joseph was eating and talking properly again within a week.

A case like Joseph's is straightforward, but sometimes hiccupping remains a complete mystery. When I was in Melbourne I met Ian, who had arrived to attend a routine appointment for which he had been waiting for some time. His wife accompanied him to the packed clinic on a sunny Thursday afternoon, and they were the picture of patience when I called them in.

When I asked Ian what the problem was, he said, 'Can't you hear it?'

'Hear what?'

He had developed hiccups in his teenage years and still had them, aged forty-five.

'So this has been going on for nearly thirty years?' I asked incredulously.

He confirmed that it had. I didn't have to take a history to work out that if he had been making this strange noise all of his adult life, then he must have married, held a job and conceived several children, hic-cupping all the way.

'Did you hiccup your way up the aisle on your wedding day?' I asked, rather rudely. I was just bowled over by how unperturbed both Ian and his wife seemed to be.

'You get used to it,' his wife said in a matter-of-fact tone. 'And, sure, is that not what love is? The good, the bad and the ugly.'

Ian could not remember the exact moment it started and said that he had woken up one day in his mid-teens and started hiccupping, and never stopped. He had seen many doctors over the years, and had had multiple tests of his lungs and stomach, but no cause was found. He was also seen by a number of psychiatrists in case there were some unresolved childhood anxiety disorder; nothing was found – he was a perfectly happy child with a loving family. Now, as a last resort, he had been sent to a neurologist. Of course, most cases of hiccups are not due to neurological disorders. Indeed, I had never seen such a case before, and have only seen a couple since.

An MRI scan revealed a small scar in the lower part of the stem of his brain. The scar was likely due to a small stroke as a teenager (most likely, but purely speculatively, caused by a tear or dissection of a blood vessel in his neck). As there was nothing that could be done to remove the scar without potentially causing untold nerve damage to the surrounding brain structures, we tried a number of medications to alleviate the symptom.

As is often the case, Ian felt the medication made him feel 'stupid' and 'like a zombie' and he decided to stop it, a reasonable thing to do in the circumstances. The hiccups returned.

There was nothing more I could do to help him. In my early days a case like this, which seemed to confirm the stereotype that neurologists 'make a diagnosis and apologize', would make me despondent. But get-ting an explanation for what had caused the hiccupping gave Ian and his wife peace of mind. They could finally stop worrying that something sinister, like a brain tumour, was growing in Ian's head. He said he was so used to the symptom he could live with it now that he was sure it was not going to kill him. 'So I am not mad, but I am *unique*,' was his happy response. He was (almost) unique. I presume he is hiccupping to this day.

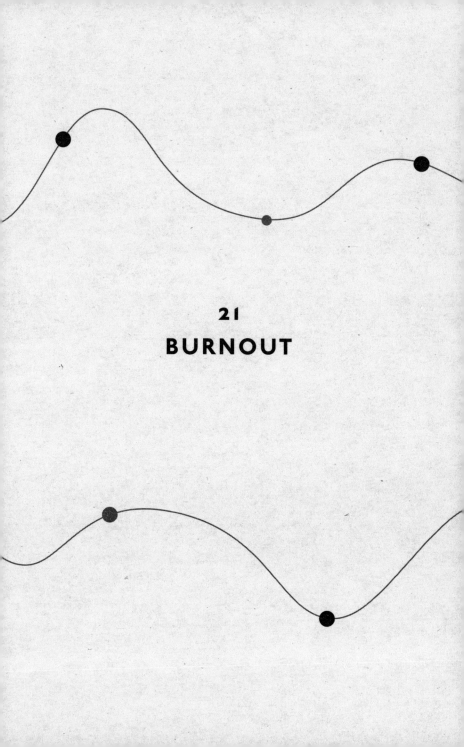

21

BURNOUT

I never really considered, until I was much older, how my father must have felt driving home from his rounds on a weekend morning, puffing furiously on a Silk Cut purple. Ireland is a small place, and it is inconceivable that he would not have been socializing with some of his patients or their relatives. These were stories you would rarely hear told in any detail, particularly because of his work with people suffering from addictions. And there was never a shortage of patients for him in 1970s and 1980s Ireland. People came from all over the country with their own stories and those of their families being torn apart by alcoholism. So he talked in general terms – how marriages were destroyed by an alcoholic spouse resistant to his attempts at therapy; the abuse suffered by the children of an alcoholic parent who refused or was unable to stop drinking; or the havoc wreaked by a drug-addicted child on their parents and siblings.

Not everyone can be helped, and I recall in my late teenage years going for my first legal pints with my father in our local village. He would go in ahead and survey the room. 'Not this one,' he would whisper, shutting the door behind him as I waited in the street. We would try one or two more pubs before he would settle on one that he deemed safe. When I asked him about this strange habit, he explained that not all patients wanted to see the doctor who had 'failed' to cure them of their alcoholism, particularly while they were drinking in their local.

Some former patients could be abusive, and he did not want to expose me to an embarrassing scene. How sad, I thought. He was doing his best to help people, but those whose treatment was not successful were actively unpleasant to him. I would come to understand in time that this was part of the downside of being a doctor, particularly if you are a local doctor, although he denied that it upset him when I asked him many years later.

I also remember sitting with him over a few pints one night when the door of the pub was thrown open by a well-known figure in Dublin at the time. He gave my father a barely perceptible nod, and walked briskly around the pub, checking every nook and cranny. He left as quickly as he had arrived, alone. 'What's he doing?' I asked.

'The poor man is probably looking for his wife,' my dad said grimly as he took a sip of his pint. 'He will probably repeat the same routine in the next four or five pubs until he finds her.' He paused briefly. 'And then he will do the same tomorrow night, and the night after that.' I knew better than to ask more.

As he got older my father seemed to withdraw socially, and preferred instead the company of a small group of people in the comfort of his own home. Obviously, this isn't unique – our circle of friends tends to diminish as we age and the vagaries of life, children, jobs take priority – but I think my father's world outside work began to shrink over time. He lived and worked in the same small area of Dublin all of his professional life and, in seeing thousands of patients from the area each year, there must have been few people left who had not either attended him as a patient themselves or been affected by someone who had. I think he just wanted to avoid any awkwardness for them or himself and so he went out less and less as time passed.

And in the end, I think, Dad fell out of love with the job of being a doctor. He was frustrated by the changes that were coming into his daily working life. The increasing need for paperwork did not appeal to him (does it appeal to anyone?), and the influence of hospital managers on doctors of his vintage was a particular bugbear. Now and again he would lament how his influence was being undermined by people many years his junior and with no medical experience at all. He kept these frustrations private but it was clear he was losing his enthusiasm for the job.

I think he also wearied of the unrelenting human suffering he had to deal with every day. He worked in the same post for thirty-odd years, and every hour of every working day he would listen to the tragic stories of those afflicted by alcoholism, by drugs, by depression and other diseases of the mind and body. Such consistent exposure to the frailties of your fellow man must be a heavy personal burden to bear, I now think. The nature of the doctor–patient relationship means that it is a burden you bear alone.

Of course, he still enjoyed some parts of his working life. I remember the occasional party when his registrars would come back to his house, singing and laughing late into the night. He liked being around the younger doctors, much like I do now. Their sense of energy and idealism is a reminder of your younger self, and the wide-eyed look of a young doctor on first witnessing a condition that you have seen many times before jolts you back to the enthusiasm of your early days. And, however he felt about his own career in his latter working years, he was proud of any achievements I might have had, especially becoming a consultant and living just up the road from the house where I had spent my medical school years under his tutelage and protection.

When it came time to retire, he did not want a retirement party or an event to mark the occasion – he was too self-conscious for the attention it would bring. I think his colleagues tried to organize some sort of celebration, but only a few days before he finally left the hospital building for the last time he had another heart attack. I was then living in Melbourne but luckily had travelled to London for a meeting so I got home quickly. It was so sad to see him in the coronary care unit, though he was upbeat as always. Because I had been qualified for many years by that stage, I felt more comfortable talking to the cardiologists about my father's prognosis than I had been that time in Galway when I had just finished pre-med.

It did not look good. Would he die while I was off in Australia? Was this the last time I would see him? Should I stay? All of these questions were going through my head, but after a few days he asked me when I was going back. I went quiet and said I was supposed to go in a few days, but that I was worried about him.

'Don't be ridiculous,' he scolded. 'You have to get on with your life, and I'll be fine.'

He was, if not quite fine, at least OK, within a few weeks, though his heart never entirely recovered. His health was a source of constant low-level anxiety and I feared that the next call from home might bring bad news. If that call were to come, I would be too far away to get back in time to say goodbye. (The fear was mainly about my father; Mum, thankfully, has always had robust good health. I'm mindful of this fear of getting bad news from home when I deal with families in work. Emigration haunts so many of the families I deal with. *Is Mum so sick that we call everyone back from America?* It can be hard to say. You don't want to be the boy who cried wolf, but nor do you want to be the one who makes the wrong call, meaning that a mother dies without her children getting home to see her one more time.)

By the time of my dad's second heart attack, our parents had been separated for nearly twenty years and Dad had met his future second wife and started a family with her. Myself and my siblings realized that this was giving him another chance at life – one I felt he thoroughly deserved after such a long period of being alone in the world. I think it also gave him the determination to stay as well as he could for his new young family and, to most of the medical people's amazement (including my own), he lived many more years to see his precious two younger daughters grow up to their late teenage years.

My father died in 2013. I still miss him. He left more of a legacy than I ever realized and his influence on my career becomes more profound with each passing year.

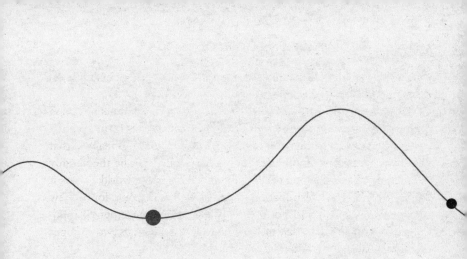

22
OFF-BALANCE

'I woke up, turned to my left to ask my husband the time, and my world turned upside down. The whole room flew past my eyes. I sat up, screamed out "help" and promptly threw up all over my husband who was still sleeping. I felt like I was on a ship being tossed about by a stormy sea, or as if I was in the worst aeroplane turbulence of my life. I was sure I was going to die. At best, I was having a stroke.'

Simone then held her vomit-soaked husband and tried to regain a sense of calm. She sat unmoving and the violent vomiting stopped briefly. When she moved her head again the vomiting became relentless. The photographs of her children flew past her and the bedside books appeared to be spinning on the table. The ambulance arrived within ten minutes and she had worked out by now that moving her head was not an option if she was not going to destroy the bedroom. The paramedics gave her an injection for the nausea and carried her from the bedroom as if they were carrying a fragile glass cabinet.

I saw her in Casualty that morning and Simone was as white as a ghost. Her vomiting had settled to a desperate retching that was only relieved by sitting stock-still. I coaxed her to stand up and to try to take a few steps. She listed to the left, for all the world like someone who had drunk a few bottles of wine ('I have not been drinking,' she managed to whisper). When she stood with her feet close together and her eyes closed she toppled over dramatically. I held my finger up in front of her eyes and when she looked to the left and right her eyes moved like the windscreen wipers on a car window when the rain is drying up. They dragged across from one side to the other, causing her immense discomfort, and this induced further retching.

She could speak, she could see, her face was symmetrical, and she was moving her arms and legs normally, so a stroke was most improbable. When I got her to walk up and down on the spot, eyes closed, her arms out in front of her like Frankenstein's monster, she quickly turned almost 180 degrees and ended up facing the opposite wall when she opened her eyes again. I got her to lie back on the trolley and held her head as I gently eased her back over the edge of the bed and turned her head one way and then the other – similar to the position you take to kiss the Blarney Stone, apparently. Turning her head to the left was fine but when I leaned her head over the bottom of the bed on her right side she threw up on the floor and her eyes appeared to be dancing in her head.

We use our ears to hear, obviously, but many people don't realize how our ears help us balance. The inner part of our ears has three little canals, called semi-circular canals, which communicate with our eyes to help keep our sense of equilibrium as we move around. This is called our vestibular, or balance, system. These fragile canals are damaged when, say, someone gets a blow to the head. I see concussed sportsmen and women who have an inner sense of unsteadiness long after they appear to have recovered from their injury. It can be hard for them to explain, but usually they agree that it is a non-specific sense of unease that they too liken to being on a ship.

So Simone had a frighteningly acute form of vertigo, known as benign paroxysmal positional vertigo, or BPPV. This is surprisingly common and quite easy to treat, but when someone develops symptoms, it's a serious shock to the system.

Simone was sure she was dying the morning that her BPPV set in. She laughed as she told me that while she lay in the ambulance, she was planning the music to be played at her funeral, and making lists in her head of whom she did and did not want to attend. Simone was very cool.

'I know you think I am being melodramatic,' – I didn't – 'but unless you have experienced that helplessness you can never really appreciate the fear.'

I have heard comments like this from patients many times and, despite having seen thousands of patients each year for many years, I still wholeheartedly agree. Try as you might, you can never wholly empathize with a sick person unless you have been sick yourself. Even then, each person's illness is different. How each individual reacts to a diagnosis is equally variable, so what seems like a benign malady to the doctor can be far from benign in its effects on a person's life, and on those around them. 'Benign' to most doctors is cause for celebration. After all, when on a daily basis you are giving some people a death sentence it is no small relief to be able to say you can actually cure someone. So a BPPV diagnosis is a good day for doctor and patient alike because the next person through the door might not be so fortunate.

The lining of one of Simone's semi-circular canals in her inner ear had come loose. The exquisitely finely tuned ebb and flow of inner-ear fluid traversing these canals now carried in it minute stones (otoconia) causing small eddy currents to the flow. This change in flow disrupted the nerve signals from her inner ears to the control centre for her eye movements when her head was held in certain positions, but not in others. It was as if the wallpaper lining the canals had peeled off and dropped into the slow-flowing water, and the disrupted flow was causing her acute vertiginous symptoms.

The solution was the weird-looking 'Epley manoeuvre', whereby the patient lies on one side and is gradually turned over, quite like a rotisserie chicken – not a very pleasant analogy, I admit, but most people get the gist. By rotating the person's head slowly, the loose 'stones' are emptied internally from the canals, restoring the normal flow of fluid.

For Simone it was just a few days before she was back to her usual self with no lingering physical or psychological effects. For others, the symptoms can grumble on for months or years, changing their entire lives. Most people have a single acute episode, get the right treatment, and get on with their lives, making it hugely satisfying to treat as a neurologist, and a massive relief to patients.

Carried away with the romance of his daughter's wedding, and a few too many celebratory drinks, Eddie decided that at sixty-eight years of age he was still able to jive the way he and his wife used to in the 1960s and he swung the light of his life enthusiastically to Bill Haley. As the 'clock struck two' he fluffed his dance move and let go of his wife, toppling backwards into a dessert trolley and finally coming to rest with a thump to the back of his head on the dance floor's edge. He jumped up quickly, profoundly embarrassed, of course, but with just a small cut to the back of his head and a massive bruise to his paternal pride.

Eddie felt fine, he insisted, but drank no more and an hour or so later made his excuses and went to his hotel room. The next morning his world too was turning upside down, as he cursed his decision to pay for the cheaper wine the wedding planner had offered. Surely it was to blame. He vomited once or twice, and after a few minutes the spinning settled into a low-grade pulsating headache with a disconcertingly persistent sense of nausea. He soldiered on through the barbeque that day, but was unable to eat the food he had paid for, and his daughter was raging with him for making a fool of himself the night before, which didn't help matters.

Over the next few weeks the symptoms settled and he put his unpleasant experience, sensibly, down to concussion rather than a prolonged hangover. But he continued to feel vaguely out of sorts for months, and decided he needed to do something about it. He had become temperamental and was acting strangely; he was starting to snap at his wife and work colleagues over minor issues that ordinarily would not have bothered him.

It is always interesting to watch how physical symptoms can affect a patient's mood and how this in turn affects their relationships. They will attribute all of their problems to, say, that fall on the dance floor, and tell anyone who will listen how it has ruined their lives. After a while, family and friends will get bored of the complaining; after all, he looks fine – no blood, no stitches, no cast; he can't be that sick. He's probably turning into a grumpy old man. (Oh, how we love our stereotypes!) As life with the sick person becomes progressively more unpleasant, people start to distance themselves, and the patient becomes isolated and depressed.

Eddie came to see me about a year after his daughter's wedding. I was his last hope, he said forlornly. He had seen any number of doctors and had at least two brain scans, but the scans were clear and he was told he had suffered a mild concussion, about which he was now understandably depressed.

I agreed with these interpretations of his symptoms but, in addition, it turned out that he had injured at least one of the semi-circular canals of the vestibular system in his ears, which explained his unease and ongoing nausea. When he was reading a book or scrolling through his phone, he felt wretched. I reproduced the symptoms he got when reading by making him move his eyes left to right, which in turn revealed the same dry-windshield-wiper effect that Simone had shown.

I arranged for him to see a physiotherapist who specialized in helping people retrain their damaged vestibular systems through a series of exercises. I reminded him that his symptoms had been present for a year, and that he should expect a slow recovery. When a rugby player breaks a leg, he does not take off the cast and run out into the Aviva stadium. He has to slowly rebuild the atrophied muscles and rehabilitate in a gradual manner to regain his former physical ability. Almost as important, a player has to regain his psychological strength after losing his sense of invincibility.

A simple injury like that having such catastrophic results enthrals me. Eddie himself marvelled at how quickly his health and self-confidence were taken away from him. It took a few months, but he gradually recovered his sense of physical and mental equilibrium. He was embarrassed by how he had reacted to what he now saw as a minor injury and apologized to everyone he had been short with. Eddie later told me that the physiotherapist had restored his sense of hope – though he swore that his jiving days were over. I wasn't convinced and I had a feeling he'd be back out there 'Dad dancing' again the next time a wedding band struck up 'Rock around the Clock'.

23
A HIDDEN SIDE OF CANCER

Tom was a twenty-year-old Gaelic footballer. His father had played before him and loved the fact that his son was following in his footsteps by playing on the Under-21 team at their local club. Tom was popular and had a wide circle of friends both in real life and online, as is the way of things these days. One November morning, he arrived downstairs to the kitchen in a state of distress. 'My phone has been hacked,' he said to his mother.

'What do you mean?' she asked.

'My Facebook page, my Twitter feed; everything has been hacked,' he said.

He was apoplectic with rage and his mother tried to calm him down. She knew things had not been quite right for the previous few weeks, but small events suddenly took on new significance. He had been involved in a row with a college mate, which was most out of character, and he had started to question his tutors aggressively during lectures. His mother had heard of these events and asked Tom whether anything was wrong. He had side-stepped her questions by explaining that he felt under pressure at college and was finding it difficult to keep up with some of his course work.

Tom was convinced now that he was the victim of an online campaign to discredit him socially, and hence his belief that his phone had been hacked. He cancelled his Facebook, Twitter and Instagram accounts. By the end of the day he seemed less agitated but the following morning his mother knew something was seriously awry when a friend of his called to ask whether he had made it home. Tom had gone with friends to the college bar, but at some point had walked out without saying where he was going. The friends had also been worried about changes in his behaviour and had gone looking for him. They found him wandering alone on the football pitch ranting about the mountains collapsing around him. They thought perhaps his drink had been spiked (he had only had two pints) and talked him out of his fugue-like state to the point where he said he was fine and was going to get a taxi home. They let him head off but remained concerned enough to call his mother the following morning.

I saw his distraught parents and his sister outside the small cubicle in Casualty later that morning. By now Tom was asleep on a trolley but he had seemingly been nonplussed earlier about why he was in hospital and why his family was so upset. A psychiatrist had been called, and had spoken with Tom and quickly concluded it was more a neurological than a psychiatric issue.

Although Tom could walk and talk he seemed to be detached from his surroundings. He answered my questions slowly and, like a phone call to Hong Kong, there seemed to be a delay between my questions and his responses. He followed my request to walk in a straight line and was able to enunciate various complex phrases I asked him to say. He was oddly incurious about what was going on. The rest of his physical examination was fine so we arranged a brain scan, which revealed a bright spot in his temporal lobes (memory centres). We also performed a lumbar puncture.

The tests confirmed he had an unusual autoimmune condition called limbic encephalitis. This is yet another condition whereby the immune system becomes over-zealous and the antibodies it produces to protect us start attacking normal tissue. These autoimmune conditions can arise spontaneously or following an infection, but they can also herald an occult cancer elsewhere in the body. That means a cancer that is already causing harmful effects, without our yet knowing where the primary tumour is. In these cases the first symptoms a person develops may be neurological – changes in personality or even seizures – arising from the antibodies attacking areas of the brain.

We checked Tom for such a cancer and found he had a small lump in his testicle that subsequently proved cancerous. Once the cancer was removed, the stimulus for the rogue antibodies that were attacking his brain would be halted. However, Tom still needed 'good antibodies' – immunoglobulins – to defeat his own 'bad antibodies' to allow the attack on his memory centres to cease.

Thankfully, Tom responded brilliantly to the treatment and within weeks he was back home and had reopened all of his social media accounts. When I met him again he had little recall of his stay in hospital or of any of our conversations during his time with us. His parents could not believe what had happened. I wondered how long it would take them to stop looking over their shoulders whenever their son behaved in any way out of the ordinary – in other words, like a typical college student.

Ophelia, better known as Hamlet's love interest in Shakespeare's play, is forced to choose between her father and brother, who warn her against the liaison and her love for the Danish prince. Slowly she descends into madness.

I had never heard of Ophelia syndrome until I met Jack when I worked in Melbourne. He was forty-three years old. When I was called to see him in the hospital's emergency department his wife described how her quiet and studious husband had changed over the preceding seven or eight months. He paid his rent several times in one day and got lost in familiar places, and this, coupled with increasingly obvious problems with his day-to-day memory, caused her to seek medical help. He was sent to see a psychiatrist, and with some anti-psychotic medication he appeared more settled for a few weeks.

This loving husband, who had rarely so much as raised his voice to his wife or children, then began to display increasingly aggressive tendencies. He was brought into the hospital by the police when they were called following an assault on his brother. How could this man who had never harmed anyone in his life suddenly undergo such an extreme change in personality?

Jack was calm when I met him but, like Tom in the previous story, bizarrely indifferent to the chaos around him. He seemed uninterested in why he was in hospital and unconcerned about the distress he was causing his family. There was no loss of muscle strength in his arms or legs and he could walk and move his eyes normally. But his speech was slurred and he found it troublesome drinking from a glass of water.

Jack also had clear-cut memory problems. We tested his cognitive abilities using the Montreal Cognitive Assessment Score. This assesses a number of cognitive abilities, including short-term memory and basic questions about the day, date and year. Jack scored fifteen out of a possible thirty.

From the rest of the neurology examination we found a right-sided palsy (or paralysis) of the tenth, eleventh and twelfth cranial nerves – those that enable us to speak and to swallow food and water. Closer examination revealed a small rubbery lump in the right side of his neck. Jack probably had some form of cancer, but how was it connected to the neurological presentation and personality change? If the cancer had spread directly to his brain surely it would have shown itself months ago?

A lumbar puncture revealed some abnormal white cells and an excess of protein that, though non-specific, indicated that whatever was causing the lump in his neck was now attacking his brain and the nerves coming from it. A scan of his upper body showed abnormal lymph nodes or glands throughout his chest and in his armpits. A brain scan showed more inflammation there. Finally, a biopsy of the rubbery lump identified that Jack had lymphoma (Hodgkin's type).

With chemotherapy Jack recovered within months but could not remember any part of his initial hospitalization. By the time he was ready for home, his cognitive score had risen to twenty-seven and his brain scan was greatly improved.

I saw him in the clinic a few months later. He came alone. Although he was, once again, living independently and working full-time, his wife had had enough and had left him and he was barred from seeing his children. Although physically he had survived cancer he was a broken man psychologically and socially.

We never found any cancer cells in his brain and we assumed that the cancer had caused his immune system to produce rogue antibodies, similar to Tom's case, but all the ones we knew of and had tested for were absent in Jack's blood and spinal fluid. The diagnosis of limbic encephalitis was similar to Tom's but we had not found the antibody to confirm it definitively in Jack's case.

One of my colleagues had been deeply involved in the case and it is to her credit that she continued to show interest many months after Jack had been discharged from hospital. She read an article in a neurology journal about Ophelia syndrome, which I had never heard of to that point. It described a new antibody that attacks the brain and can appear, very rarely, in people with Hodgkin's lymphoma. We tested some of Jack's spinal fluid from the time of his original presentation in Casualty and to our astonishment it proved to be positive for these antibodies.

Jack's cancer had been insidiously over-stimulating his own immune system, causing personality and memory changes many months before the cancer itself became apparent. He had descended, temporarily, into a Shakespearean form of madness.

24
ANTHONY'S STORY

Anthony stepped out of his car, caught his foot in the car door frame and crashed on to the wet pavement outside his home. He cut his forehead badly on the concrete and was bleeding profusely from his left hand when he came into the kitchen.

His wife gasped. 'Were you in a fight?'

'I just slipped getting out of the car,' he said, embarrassed, his pride more injured than anything else.

Looking back later, Anthony knew this was the moment when he had become sick. Over the following weeks, it became evident to him that his left hand was slow to heal. His grip on the steering wheel was off – perhaps he had done more damage in the fall than he had thought – but he ignored it. He assumed he had sprained his wrist and things would settle.

After a month, his hand was cramping when he lay in bed at night, and he found it a handicap at his work as a carpenter. A left-hander, he couldn't seem to use his drill as adroitly as he did before and began to worry he may have damaged the nerves in his hand. He decided to see his doctor soon, but kept putting it off.

'Too busy,' he explained to me later. 'Work is insane at the moment and, as I am self-employed, I cannot afford to turn down any jobs. I didn't have the time to arrange an appointment.'

He had never been one for doctors anyway, and didn't want to waste his time or money seeing a doctor who would only tell him what he knew already: that he had sprained his hand and it just needed some anti-inflammatories and rest (and the latter wasn't going to happen). He carried on as usual and bought some strapping in Boots to form a makeshift splint for his sprained wrist and hand. He started applying some gels to ease the cramps and took Nurofen at night to ease the pain.

He nearly seriously injured his apprentice some weeks later when he dropped the drill on the poor guy's foot. That did it. As soon as he finished that job, he booked an appointment with his GP. His arm had been 'complaining to him', he said. What he meant was not that it was bothering him, but that when he took off his splint, he could see the muscles in his forearm rolling around spontaneously 'like they were waving at me, trying to get my attention'.

His GP arranged x-rays and an appointment with an orthopaedic surgeon. 'Probably just a sprain,' the surgeon agreed, and the x-rays showed nothing had been broken. He thought it likely the weakness of grip was due to pain, so, as Anthony had predicted, he was told to take anti-inflammatories and rest the arm as much as he could. He was also scheduled for a physiotherapy session: 'fecking useless' was his judgement, and after three sessions he abandoned the exercises.

As his hand got weaker, Anthony realized that something was seriously wrong. He didn't tell his wife. Put off by his first experience with the doctor, he started googling 'arthritis' and 'nerve damage'. He convinced himself he had a variety of medical conditions – carpal tunnel syndrome; repetitive strain injury; and even early rheumatoid arthritis. Meanwhile, his hand was undeniably getting weaker, and he had been forced to adapt his drilling technique at work. He started driving his car almost entirely using his right hand. Three months after he had fallen from his car he tripped again. He had been focused on his useless left hand, but suddenly realized that his left leg was weak too. He panicked – 'I must be having a stroke' – and drove himself to Casualty.

Anthony sat in a room on his own, listening to the comings and goings of Casualty outside. He hadn't told anyone else he was coming. The very act of coming to the hospital had nearly broken him. All of his attempts at denying that something serious might be wrong had folded as soon as the nurse saw him. She knew instantly that his symptoms were ominous, and fast-tracked him on to a trolley. He had then seen a young doctor, who noted the 'waving muscles' in his arms and also knew this was not going to end well. The young doctor explained that Anthony's symptoms did not appear to be related to his joints but were due to a nerve problem. Then I was called in.

I knocked on the door. 'Come in,' he whispered. Tears streamed down his face as he sat scrolling through his phone. Most people do not know the difference between a neurologist and a neurosurgeon, so my patients are often frightened to see me, thinking that they're about to be wheeled off to brain surgery. When I explain that neurologists listen to patients' stories, examine them and order tests, as relieved as they might be, they probably think that sounds pretty useless by comparison to surgery.

He composed himself, and I listened to his story. He had admitted to himself that the fall from his car was a symptom, not the cause of his weak left hand. He had begun to notice his left leg following suit. His voice was shaking and, at times, I could sense the excess of saliva at the back of his throat. He saw me looking, and jumped in with, '– and I can't seem to stop all this spit building up! It's so embarrassing. I carry boxes of tissues with me to avoid looking like a dribbling mess.'

As we talked, it came out that he had four young children, and he showed me a photograph of them all together at the foot of the Sugar-loaf mountain, where they went for family picnics in the summer months. I knew the area well, and recalled many years of my own family doing the same thing. He stood up so that I could examine his gait, and we could both hear the slap of his left foot on the floor. The cap of his left work boot was scuffed and worn down. This had clearly been going on for months, and he pointed out that he would catch the foot on cracked pavements and was tripping on the stairs all the time unless he concentrated. 'I never thought I would have to think about climbing the stairs,' he told me. He was only forty-six years old.

He took off his T-shirt and we both looked at the undulating muscles in his arms and all over his chest. This is what he meant when he described his muscles waving at him. These 'fasciculations' are invari-ably a bad omen. The nerves supplying the 'electricity' to the muscles were failing throughout his body, and I could see the rippling tissue in his legs, his arms and even on his tongue. This burly man now had vis-ibly atrophied muscles in his hands, which looked like they belonged to a much older and frailer man. He could not even grip the piece of paper I proffered to test his dexterity.

This was the beginning of the end for poor Anthony, I thought to myself. He could recognize it in my eyes, seeing through my attempts to hide my concern for him. 'How bad, Doc?' he asked. 'I really need to know. I have to look after my wife, my kids, the business, the mortgage . . . everything.' My heart broke for him. I knew it was doubt-ful that Anthony would be alive a year from now.

One might think that all the worries of life would dissolve into insignificance at moments like this, but the practical nature of people astounds me. He had hardly talked about himself and his own fears at all; he just wanted to make sure that his family was going to be OK. We went on with the exam. His reflexes were brisk despite his failing nerves. 'At least that's a good sign, right?' he asked hopefully. I scratched the soles of his feet and both of his big toes sprung upwards. None of these were good signs at all.

Motor neuron disease had been much in the news as the bogey-man of all neurological conditions and it is the worst nightmare of all neurologists. As a diagnosis, it is a death sentence, but the condition can vary in terms of how aggressive it is. Typically, patients have a year of symptoms before a diagnosis is made, and then it is a year or two until death, but I have seen people live for years with this cruel condition and battle grimly in the face of the loss of control of their arms, their legs and eventually their speech and ability to swallow.

When and where do you tell someone they are going to die? Is it in a side room of Casualty, when they're alone? Should you make it more obvious by asking them to call their loved ones in, and explain it to them when they are all together? Do you gently hint at a diagnosis over a few days? Or end the misery of the patient's not knowing and risk seeming cruel by getting straight to the point?

Of course, there is no right or wrong answer, no manual. You just have to try to judge each case on its own merits and hope you get it right – or at least not horrendously wrong. Anthony was smart and, though very upset, he wasn't angry. What he wanted were answers, immediately. There are some conditions that mimic motor neuron disease, and that are treatable. As a result, I would never say straight out that a patient had motor neuron disease until I had exhausted all the other possibilities. This involves getting blood tests, electrical tests of the muscles and MRI scans. The tests serve to make sure I am not fooled by an unusual presentation of some other rare condition.

I told Anthony that I was worried about a number of conditions – sometimes a white lie is kinder than the blunt truth when you have not yet confirmed a diagnosis. It may seem unfair but it would have been worse, I think, if you told someone they had an incurable disease before investigating thoroughly.

This time, though, the tests would only confirm what I already knew. I described how the nerves or wires to his muscles were failing.

'Like a dodgy light switch?' he asked. 'Well, who is the electrician and how can we get him to fix the switch?'

I outlined the tests we would do and that he should plan to stay in the hospital to speed up a diagnosis. 'I haven't time for that,' he replied. 'I have a communion and a confirmation this weekend; I have two big jobs on at the moment. I don't have the time to be sitting around hospitals. Will it be quicker if I pay for the tests?' he asked.

'No. It's not a question of money, but one of time. We need you to stay in hospital and get everything done smartly so we can plan ahead if there are any treatments for you.'

And there it was. *If.*

'What do you mean, "if"? What is this "if"? Are you saying there might be a chance this is *not* treatable? Do you think I have cancer?'

His voice had risen an octave. Before my eyes I watched him grapple with his own mortality, all in an instant. He was both heartbroken and terrified.

'I am worried,' I said reluctantly, 'that you might have motor neuron disease.' I paused.

The tears rolled down his cheeks and he said nothing.

I went on. 'There are other conditions that look a lot like motor neuron disease and *are* treatable, so I am asking you to stay in the hospital so that we can look for all treatable alternatives.'

'But what about the communion? The confirmation? The kids will be in bits if I'm not there,' he said. He'd returned to worrying about everyone else again – it's a lot easier to do, in a way.

'You can still go out to both,' I told him, 'but you will just have to come back to the hospital afterwards while we work this all out.'

'Jesus,' he exclaimed as the gravity of what was confronting him began to sink in. 'Motor neuron is that one with the ice buckets, isn't it? No one survives that, do they?'

★

While Anthony was being admitted, I went on to see the other patients who had come in through Casualty that day: a young girl with migraine; an old woman who had suffered a mini-stroke; a worried mother with a shaking hand; and a 32-year-old man with dizzy spells. Then I dropped back to see Anthony. He wasn't on the neurology ward. The nurse told me he had gone out for a cigarette. 'He has been on the phone constantly since you left,' she said.

I went out to the hospital entrance, where he was talking animatedly into his phone. 'It's going to be fine,' he was saying. 'They just want to do some tests. I will be at the communion on Saturday, so don't worry. But better bring me in some pyjamas and slippers if I have to stay in this kip.' He caught my eye as he said this and tried to hide his cigarette by cupping it in his hand. Smoking is the least of your worries right now, I thought, as I waved him over.

'How are you feeling?' I asked, rather uselessly.

'Well, Doc, it is what it is,' he smiled grimly. 'Let's just get on with the tests and see how it goes. I've been sorting out the jobs at work so they're covered for this week. The wife will be in later after the school runs. Life goes on, doesn't it?'

It was just hours since I had suggested the diagnosis, and he was almost buoyant.

'We are going to fight this thing, aren't we?' he said.

As doctors we can fool ourselves into thinking that someone is coming to terms with their illness. It certainly makes it easier to deal with for the doctors and nurses looking after people if they seem to have somehow made peace with where they find themselves. That's because, with terminal diagnoses, the futility of much of our work is never far from our thoughts. We do an awful lot of good and cure the majority of those we see, but there are times when modern medicine is still no match for an illness. And motor neuron disease is one of those illnesses.

I smiled and agreed that, of course, we would fight it all the way. What else could I say?

Over the following week I saw Anthony at least twice a day. He was the life and soul of the ward, where he organized an evening card game. I would catch him off guard sometimes wandering back to the ward on his own from his daily smokes – 'I promise, I am cutting down – I just need a few each day to help the stress of all this,' he'd explain bashfully.

The hospital must feel like a prison at times. Your day is ordered for you. You are woken for breakfast and pills. You are called for tests and therapies. You watch the doctors and nurses arrive in an entourage each day and discuss your progress. You observe the medical students unable to hide their emotions at your diagnosis. You are away from all the comforts of home and your loved ones. When they do visit, they come in with heads tilted and awkward conversation ensues. Their daily news of who did what at school or who called around to the house must seem extraordinarily mundane, compared with what you're facing, so visits can be trying for everyone, though patients are lost without them. You make friends (and indeed enemies) among your fellow patients – the camaraderie that develops can be wonderful – and then watch as some head home having been given the all-clear. *When will it be my turn to go home? When does my sentence end?* For some, it doesn't.

It is beyond sobering for longer-term patients when one of their circle dies on the other side of the curtain opposite them, surrounded by an army of doctors trying and failing to revive them. The next day someone new will have moved into the recently vacated bed. No one talks about the events of the night before, as it's all too close for comfort. A silent breakfast follows. The daily routine resumes and by nightfall there is someone new at the card table who never asks how they gained their place there.

A week or so on, and Anthony had had his scans, electrical tests and therapy. 'She may be a sergeant major, but I am definitely feeling the strength back in my hands,' Anthony told me of the physio, delighted with the success of his therapy sessions. I walked with him to the side room with his wife, whom I had asked to come in. They already knew the result in their hearts. From this moment, they couldn't deny it any longer.

'The tests confirm what we were most worried about,' I explained. 'You have motor neuron disease.' During his week in hospital, Anthony had convinced himself that things would be OK.

His wife burst into tears and started shouting, 'No, no. You must be wrong!' Anthony took her hand. 'I don't think he is, love,' he said. 'Can I go home now, Doc?' he asked. 'Is there anything else we can do?'

I always arrange a second opinion when it comes to motor neuron disease. There is always an outside possibility that we are wrong. It also gives people time to process what is happening, and to generate the myriad questions they will have but are too shell-shocked to ask when you tell them the grim news. I explained this to Anthony and his wife.

'What's the point?' he asked. They packed up his belongings and said goodbye to his fellow 'inmates'. He didn't tell them his news, but I think they knew.

'You lucky bastard,' they joked. 'We are still stuck here in Shaw-shank, and you get to go home.' He laughed along with them and headed to the door.

I received a letter from the specialist motor neuron disease clinic a couple of months later. They could not find an alternative diagnosis for Anthony and confirmed our worst fears for him. In the meantime he had enrolled in a trial in the motor neuron clinic run by one of my colleagues with a new experimental therapy and had begun to raise funds for their research. Not everyone qualifies for such trials, and some studies that are ongoing are aimed at looking at tests that might improve our medical knowledge of the condition, but do not involve therapies. He was definitely 'fighting this', as he promised he would.

He came back to see me again just before Christmas of the same year. He was in a terrible state and now needed a wheelchair. His slurred speech was hard to make out and his wife acted as our interpreter most of the time. The box of tissues beside him attested to his inability to swallow his own saliva. He did not want to be resuscitated if he had a cardiac arrest, he said.

'They have all suffered enough,' he said, nodding towards his wife. 'I don't want them to go through any more pain.' He was still only think-ing of others, and it was incredibly heart-wrenching.

Living with a terminal neurological disease is harrowing for both patients and their families towards the end of life. There is no hiding from the slowing gait, deteriorating speech and loss of autonomy. It is awful to witness as a doctor, so I cannot imagine the toll it takes on a partner or children.

In addition, a diagnosis of motor neuron disease brings a lifetime of anxiety for the patient's survivors: although MND is only rarely genetic, how can they not worry that they are going to meet the same fate if their hand is numb when they wake up, or if they drop a plate while serving dinner? The family history of illnesses is critical, not just for determining whether or not someone may have a predisposition to a certain disease, but also in working out what the patient is most concerned about – even if they do not admit to it.

'Thanks for everything, Doc,' Anthony said as he manoeuvred his electric wheelchair out of the clinic. 'You did your best. I don't envy you your job, though.'

'Jesus', I thought, 'how can he possibly feel sorry for me?'

Anthony died in the hospice a month later surrounded by his family and many friends.

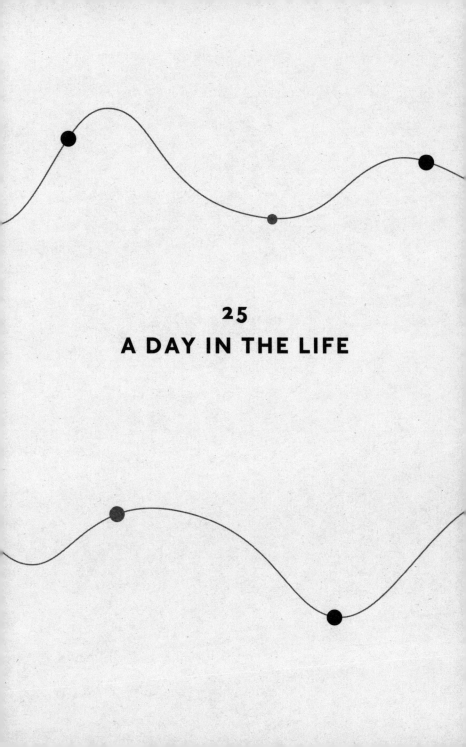

25
A DAY IN THE LIFE

I thought the Sunday night 'back to school feeling' would get better with age, but apparently it doesn't. In fact, I suspect it's getting worse. I like to get in to work early so that I can get thirty minutes alone to deal with paperwork and email referrals. Then at eight on Monday morning the team meets to go over the x-rays and brain scans of the interesting and difficult cases of the previous week or those of patients due in later that week. There are about twenty of us in this meeting – neurology consultants and students as well as doctors from other departments. We share ideas and suggest treatment options so it is very useful as a teaching forum, and patients benefit hugely from multiple doctors viewing their images and coming up with the best options available for them. Straight afterwards we have a very brief roll-call meeting of the neurology team – as you rarely know which staff members are on leave of one type or another – and by the end of the meeting we have a picture of what is happening and who is assigned to do what for the week ahead.

After that, at about 8.45 a.m. I head to Casualty (now called the Emergency Department, or ED, but I still use the old-fashioned term). With the weekend backlog, the referrals from the department trolleys come in thick and fast on a Monday morning. The state of Casualty departments – particularly at the height of winter – is a running theme of media coverage of the health service. Sometimes what reporting of the 'trolley crisis' misses, I think, is the frenetic activity in our Casualty and Acute Medical Units that goes on all the time, including at weekends. I have to say, in hospitals' defence, that the spirit of collegiality and mutual respect between doctors and nurses under extreme pressure, with the lives of so many people depending on them, is admirable. It can indeed be terribly tough for patients, but many will comment on how observing the events of a single night in one of our Casualties makes them appreciate their own lives so much more.

First, I see a 56-year-old woman with a three-stone weight loss in the previous three months. She was recently discharged from another hospital. At 4 a.m. her husband was woken by what he felt was her heavy breathing but decided it was nothing untoward and fell back asleep. By 6.30, she was unrousable, and by the time I saw her at 8.45 she was intubated and ventilated – being kept alive by artificial means. She had probably had a heart attack some hours before, and thus there was little hope of her making a meaningful neurological recovery. Her nicotine-stained hands were small and thin and there was wasting of the muscles. This suggested the possibility of an underlying cancer so it may have been better for her to have died peacefully at home in her bed.

From this resuscitation area, I go to the main Casualty, where people lie in various states of distress on trolleys. I see a sixty-year-old man with a possible stroke. His right arm is weak, he tells me, but when I examine him I cannot detect any deficit – the implication of there being no abnormal neurological signs is that he is another of the worried well. That said, to be certain, he still needs a CT brain scan. Fortunately for him, when the scan comes back it's clear and he can go home.

Next is a 68-year-old woman with severe headaches. They are likely due to occipital neuralgia (a painful nerve condition affecting a specific area on the side of the scalp) and not as serious as she fears. Across the room, a 21-year-old girl has a weak left arm. Her first cousin has MS and, understandably, this is worrying her. Again, I feel she is one of the worried well, but sending her home without an MRI scan would be indefensible, so I have to admit her. The scan usually takes place after two to three days of hospitalization because of the long list of other people already waiting for similar scans. It could be done as an outpatient but the waiting times for an outpatient scan are too prohibitively long to take the chance. I understand why someone would rather wait for days in a hospital, with disturbed sleep and variable food, than go home still in limbo as to what is wrong with them. There is no doubt in my mind, however, that many would not need to stay in hospital if we had sufficient access to urgent scans – but that is another story.

I then telephone two GPs about letters they have sent me concerning shared patients. A quick phone call to a colleague can prevent someone having to come to Casualty but will never appear on the 'metrics' that assess what doctors do so regularly.

I visit a ninety-year-old patient of mine with Parkinson's disease who fell at home and fractured his hip. He is in the geriatric ward. A courtesy call can mean so much that the extra time taken to reassure him that he is not alone or forgotten lifts both our spirits.

I move on to the Coronary Care Unit (CCU), where a 48-year-old Chinese man had been referred to me with new left arm and leg weakness (hemiparesis). 'He is on methadone,' whispers the CCU nurse. I ask her if the man under her care has any heart problems (he is, after all, in the CCU).

'No, they suspect a stroke', she says.

A young doctor in training beside her overhears and points out that the man's ECG and blood tests indicate a recent heart attack. The nurse is unabashed and informs us that those findings could indeed be in keeping with a myocardial infarction (heart attack). In fact the man has had both a stroke and a heart attack around the same time. As we walk away the young doctor rolls her eyes.

So young and already so cynical! She will learn quickly enough, I hope, about the imperfections of our craft and how even experienced people, like the CCU nurse, can be thrown by someone turning up with two serious problems at the same time.

We make a treatment plan for the poor man and then set off for the Acute Medical Unit (AMU). This is a relatively new part of the hospital set-up and serves as a sort of step-down area from Casualty, where people get a proper bed, instead of a trolley, and are assessed by an expert team of medics to determine the tests and treatments they will need while in hospital. The AMU doctors tell us that there are no neurology referrals to be seen, as we had already seen the acute cases due their way earlier in Casualty. This is fairly unusual as most days we see people in both departments.

It's about 11.30 now and I have coffee with colleagues before going to the ward where the neurology inpatients are based. We are about to go around and review all of our patients but, before we do, we go through each patient's potential problems and make sure we are clear about our plans for treatments. The registrar has been with us a year and should know what is expected of him, but he does not seem to know much about any of the patients we are about to see. I am frustrated, as this is his main job, and I let him know that I am disappointed in how he has come on in the last twelve months. While he is a good guy, he has delusions of grandeur. Sensible junior doctors are aware of their limitations, and know that with a basic six-year medical degree they are very much still on the beginner slopes. But a minority – this registrar among their number – cannot resist trying to impress patients with an air of expertise and authority. I cannot bear young doctors pretending to patients that they are better than they are. Of course, my real frustration is at what I perceive to be a lack of curiosity about all things neurological. I speak to him bluntly and I see him become flushed. Almost immediately I am filled with remorse as I recall my own inadequacies at his age. I ask him to pop in to me later and I promise myself to make amends then.

For many years I would just grab a sandwich and eat at my desk around lunchtime. A recent development has been a much more sociable lunch with colleagues in the hospital canteen. A mixed group of old and young consultants, I now lie among the former but enjoy tremendously the company of both. It is great to chat through our mutual frustrations for half an hour each day, and we try to outdo one another about which of us has had the worst day so far. Regardless of speciality, the highs and lows are similar, so it is terrific to be reminded we are not alone.

After more phone calls to patients, relatives and GPs, dictation of letters and writing updated prescriptions to be sent out to patients, I start the most difficult clinic of the week: outpatients.

First, I see a 43-year-old dentist with mild and well-controlled (by medication) epilepsy, and then a seventy-year-old woman with Parkinson's disease, followed by a 63-year-old man with the same condition. All three patients are relatively well but a five-minute reassurance consultation is impossible as each is dealing with the emotional, more than the physical, consequences of the disease labels they are stuck with for the rest of their lives.

The fourth patient is an 81-year-old man with very mild Parkinson's. Again, the 'label' of Parkinson's seems to have caused more illness than the mild tremor he actually has. A long conversation ensues and, although in truth I make no changes to his medication, with reassurance he seems less tremulous leaving than when he arrived.

Next is a 58-year-old woman who is on a blood thinner (warfarin) to prevent strokes. She has a rare condition called anti-phospholipid syndrome that can damage the blood vessels throughout the body, but she is also very well, thankfully. She's a very kind woman and it's cheering to have an upbeat conversation with a patient for the first time that day. We discuss her hobbies, she recommends some of her favourite books, and I am intrigued, as always, by how some people wear their disease labels with such equanimity while others fall apart.

I then call in a young Korean woman who has headaches. Her English isn't great, but she's very affable, and together we work out, over the course of half an hour, that she has migraine. Another half an hour is spent diagnosing a thirty-year-old Iron Man participant with MS. His father is a patient of mine and has had the same condition for over thirty years. The son's only symptom was a heavy left leg and this would develop after he ran five miles. A lengthy discussion followed about Uhthoff's phenomenon to explain his symptoms: his body appears fine when not stressed but when its temperature rises with exercise, the vulnerable parts of the nerves are exposed. The insulation – or myelin sheaths – surrounding the nerves is damaged by MS, and so conduction along the nerves to his legs is slowed by the heat generated by his running to the point that he can hardly walk at all after the sixth mile. I try to explain things without jargon, but fatigue is starting to set in. Mine isn't a long day to many people, but huge concentration is required for every consultation, and meetings with patients and their families can be emotionally fraught and take their toll.

A 29-year-old speech therapist is next and both of her parents – but, perhaps notably, not her fiancé – ask a litany of questions. She has had very mild MS for over four years and did not get on well with her previous neurologists. When seeking a second opinion, such patients are usually extremely well informed about their condition and treatment options but on this occasion it's as if I am telling them all about MS for the first time. Forty-five minutes passes very slowly indeed. I realize I have assumed too much at the start of the consultation and spoke about MS as if they all knew a lot about the condition. So I find myself going back to the very basics. I have learned yet another lesson about taking for granted what someone does or does not know about their illness.

The final patient in the clinic is a 62-year-old schoolteacher who a year before developed a twitch in his left eye when out in the playground at lunchtime. He went to an optician who terrified him by suggesting he might have a brain tumour. Like his GP, I feel this poor man has ocular migraine. A long discussion follows as he wishes to understand the mechanism of migraine at a cellular level. I don't think he is particularly satisfied with my attempts to explain it to him. I am not sure I am particularly satisfied with my efforts either.

When I finish the clinic I call the neurology registrar to check on any patients who have been referred from Casualty or the AMU while I was seeing the outpatients. There is a young woman on a trolley who the registrar is worried might have had a stroke. 'She is right-handed, dysphasic and unable to move her left side,' he explains authoritatively. A right-handed person nearly always has their speech centre on the left side of the brain. Thus, if they have difficulty speaking (are dysphasic), a stroke would affect the left side of their brain. If you have a stroke in the left side of your brain, the right side of your body will be weak. What the doctor has described does not fit with the known circuitry.

I am taken aback that I have to explain to the registrar the basics of right-handed people being left-cerebral-hemisphere-dominant, and thus he is presenting me with a neurological near impossibility. Maybe our earlier encounter has made him nervous and he has got flustered and muddled some of the rudimentary principles of neurology. When we meet later I will have to make an effort to get the feedback right. Giving feedback well is something of a challenge for me – if I could apply the same care to communicating with junior doctors as I do to communicating with patients, I'd be better at it. But when mental reserves are low, diplomacy can suffer. The registrar needs to be on top of the basics, and he needs to be robust enough not to crumble when mistakes or shortcomings are pointed out. But I need to figure out how to build his confidence and bring out the best in him.

Another elderly man has been referred by another medical team with possible early Parkinson's disease, but a quick overview of the correct medical history revealed this too is an impossibility. The younger doctors are just not bothering any more, I feel, knowing a senior neurologist will see the patient quickly regardless. It's late in the afternoon and I'm obviously running low on patience.

I check in with the neurology ward sister and as we chat I am gratified to see a 29-year-old woman with cerebral venous thrombosis, who
was drowsy and vomiting the week before, now talking normally with
her relieved fiancé. She had suffered a clot in the veins of the brain, like
those you see in the legs of some people after long-haul flights, associated with taking the contraceptive pill. He recognizes me but she, of
course, does not. We share a wry smile at her loss of recall of all the
life-threatening events of the previous week.

Back at my desk, I start to do some paperwork. The registrar knocks
on the door tentatively and comes in for a chat. He expresses his frustrations at my high expectations of him. I tell him – and I believe – that he
is right and I was wrong earlier: I *was* expecting too much. I apologize
and try to be as encouraging as I can about the things he is doing right.
(Things improve considerably in the subsequent months.)

I finish my paperwork and clear the post for the day. I finally get
home and am relieved to at last have some time alone. I don't know
how other doctors come back to chaotic families, children and meal-
times. I need time alone to decompress. I still have to get some food,
but rarely feel hungry after such an intensely draining day as the knot
in my stomach can sometimes take a few hours to untangle. I write my
diary for the following day, plan my meetings for the morning and drink
a glass of wine. I am done.

At 4 a.m., I wake spontaneously and for no apparent reason. The
patients of the previous day turn over in my mind and I wonder
whether the woman, who twenty-four hours before had woken her
husband with her heavy breathing pattern, is still alive now. She wasn't
that much older than me and in a few months she had travelled from
the land of the well to the threshold of the great abyss.

In this gloomy state, I recall two other patients I had seen the day
before. A 78-year-old woman arrived nervously with her daughter. Her
83-year-old sister had Parkinson's and she was worried that her own
tremor heralded a similar fate for herself. Fortunately, hers was an inten-
tion tremor, worse with movements such as holding a cup of tea, rather
than the resting tremor typical of Parkinson's. She and her daughter
shed a tear when I explained that she did not have her sister's condition.
A lovely moment among the horrors of bleak diagnoses that day.

Another sad but beautiful moment comes back to me. Anneka is a Dutch woman who has been a patient of mine for over ten years with a variety of ailments – migraine, minor seizures, joint pains and dizzy spells. A retired postmistress, Anneka smokes heavily and her make-up evokes images of Bette Davis in *Whatever Happened to Baby Jane?*. We always get on well and I think she enjoys her visits, more to combat loneliness than to discuss her medical problems.

Anneka had come in the previous day because her headaches had escalated in frequency and severity and the medication didn't seem to be effective any more. As we discussed possible alternatives, the usually phlegmatic Anneka asked whether I felt that stress could be playing a role in her increasingly severe headaches – 'explosions' of pain that put her out of action for days on end. She went on to explain that she had been in love with a woman in her native Holland for over forty years. She was still alive and her family had put her in a nursing home as they had felt she was suffering from dementia. Anneka disagreed. She visited her as often as she could but the family had always suspected them of an affair and had resented poor Anneka all her life.

The affair, in fact, had never been consummated and she welled up with regret about this. I asked her whether, at seventy-eight years of age, looking back now, she felt she should have taken the risk of the opprobrium of her own family, the woman's family and society in general by going ahead with the affair.

She paused and said, 'Yes, I wish I had gone for it but now it is too late.'

After a moment she said, 'Besides, Sister Lotte, who loved me then and still loves me now, could never have faced the eternal shame she would have felt at breaking her religious vows.'

Anneka's headaches were a result of her unfulfilled love. At times, the simple humanity behind neurological symptoms would break your heart.

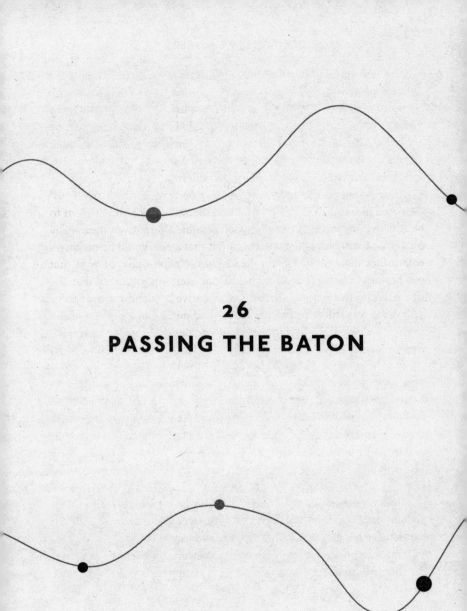

26

PASSING THE BATON

I have been teaching since I was a junior registrar but I still sometimes get nervous when about to teach a new class of students. However, once I pick up on the atmosphere of the lecture theatre or bedside teaching group, and gauge the students' level of enthusiasm, if not immediately their aptitude, for neurology, I relax and begin to enjoy the sessions. In the past I probably relaxed too much, as one of my former bosses told me. I shudder now to think of the effects some more acerbic off-the-cuff comments might have had during my earlier teaching career, usually made when coming into the lecture theatre after a difficult morning in the outpatient clinic. I am also mindful that these days students can be offended by throwaway comments that in years past would have been viewed as a professor's eccentricities. We are all learning to be more sensitive – and that is probably no harm.

A lecturer's mood and enthusiasm can be as fickle as those of the class they are trying to teach, but there is a real sense of satisfaction when you walk away from a class feeling that you have done a good job – and a sense of despondency when you don't.

Neurophobia, or fear of studying neurology, makes teaching the subject an additional challenge. This is a recognized condition that I have studied in recent years. Both medical students and non-neurology doctors find neurology difficult from their earliest years in medicine and can develop an attitude that it's too difficult to even try overcoming their fear, or that there are too many unknowns for study to be rewarding. I understand this, of course, because I found it hard going for years, and as soon as I get cocky I come across a case that confounds me and where I get a kick in the backside and realize how tricky it must seem to doctors not seeing neurology patients every day.

The fact that you cannot see or hear the brain – while you can listen to someone's heartbeat, feel their pulse, observe the veins in their necks – is certainly a drawback for some. However, I find the unknowns enthralling. There is still so much about the brain we do not know that I cannot see how anyone could not be interested in this area of medicine, and I have always loved teaching students about how much fun neurology can be.

We can take extraordinary pictures of the brain with MRI scans. We can perform electrical tests of the nerves and muscles throughout the body with neurophysiology. We can even test the fluid within which the brain and nerves are bathing with a lumbar puncture. These are vital ancillary tests of nerve and brain function. But for almost 150 years the neurological history and examination are still of the greatest importance when dealing with people with neurological problems. To my mind it is this beautifully human aspect of neurology that underpins the elegance of the subject.

Neurology lends itself to teaching through a combination of science and theatre. But, for me, getting the patient's story is central. I teach students the importance of approaching it like a detective, adopting a Sherlock Holmesian strategy to finding out the background history and making the connections. I explain the vital importance of tracing the patient's movements and habits in the lead-up to the moment they discerned something was wrong. It is like a jigsaw, and even pieces that appear dull at the outset can be as important as any other piece when we come to see the whole picture. They should keep probing, Columbo-style, until they are satisfied that they have found out as much as possible – there is always 'Just one more question . . .'

I have always enjoyed watching the students' reaction to seeing the neurology exam being performed. Explaining the mechanics of the brain and translating how we see, hear, walk and talk at a fairly basic level is wonderful fun and always thought-provoking. There may be somewhere between 150 and 200 students in the class. We have real neurology patients who have volunteered for the sessions come to the lecture theatre and I demonstrate the basics of each part of the examination. I stress that communication is everything, and physical communication in the form of mimicry is especially useful. Showing the patient the movements you wish to elicit is much more productive than merely asking them to perform each of the tasks involved. When I ask them to raise their eyebrows ('as if surprised'), or frown ('as if angry'), while doing so myself, they mirror my expressions much more easily than if I make the same requests with an expressionless face. (It can backfire when it becomes so clear to the patient that, for example, one reflex is behaving differently to another, and they quickly realize something may be truly amiss.)

I try to involve the class as much as possible, which means that I bring up individual students to have a go at doing whatever I've demonstrated. I just pick randomly from the class. While this might seem cruel, and certainly anxiety-inducing, watching a peer do a good job inspires everyone else to raise their game. And if someone does make a hash of things, then everyone feels a bit better about themselves (except the poor soul who has been put on the spot – but even they will learn from their failure, I always hope). Patients who volunteer for these educational sessions are generally good sports and their insights into their conditions humanize things for students.

Once students have the basics of taking a history and performing a competent neurology exam, we can move on to the far more captivating subject of the ways the nervous system can fail.

In teaching junior doctors how to deal with everything that will be coming at them on a daily basis I try to zero in on the most fundamental aspect of being a doctor: their relationship with their patients. Surprisingly, that includes some thoughts on etiquette and presentation. I draw the analogy with *First Dates*. First impressions are crucial. You won't make it to dessert if you eat with your mouth open, hold your utensils like weapons or look like you got dressed in the dark. And many patients don't think any differently about a doctor who looks unkempt or has poor manners.

My opening comments to final-year medical students usually involve suggestions on bedside manners. Year on year this appears to be more necessary, as students encountering a patient for the first time will simply start barking instructions at them without any explanation as to who they are, what they are doing and why they are doing it. Maybe it is a lack of confidence, or even a dearth of social skills inspired by smartphone isolation, but now it is necessary to explain to twenty-somethings that they should introduce themselves to strangers by shaking hands and saying their name.

Over the years I've heard people say that patients do not care how their doctors look as long as they are competent, but in my experience this is untrue. Patients see the seemingly superficial things and judge straight away; they've told me as much. In fact, my non-medical friends frequently comment on their doctor's appearance before thinking to mention why they went to see the doctor. First dates indeed.

And, of course, your shoes. Always with the shoes. As a medical student and younger doctor, what I wore was not very important when it came to spending whatever money I had. We were not paid much in those days and, living away from home, most of what we earned would immediately disappear on rent. If I am honest, I did not really think about it, as the priorities in those days were Tube fare and beer money. It was in London that a patient commented that I should learn how to knot a tie properly and perhaps consider polishing my cheap shoes. I was taken aback but started to notice that after each introduction most patients looked me in the eye, but immediately dropped their gaze to my shoes. And as the neurology exam starts with examining gait, naturally patients look down at your shoes when you are explaining what you would like them to do. The disappointment (or disgust) on their faces is rarely well disguised if the shoes are badly kept. (Mind you, a taste for nice shoes can go down badly if patients perceive them to be too expensive.)

So I ask students to consider the impact that their appearance, demeanour and bearing will have on the vulnerable patients in front of them. I stress how quickly trust is lost on first impressions and how difficult it is to regain. I ask them to reflect on how their parents would look upon a young doctor who had barely bothered to disguise the previous night's partying. With the female students I can be on tricky ground, as how can a fusty professor sound anything other than misogynistic (or, worse still, prurient) when suggesting that revealing clothing is best avoided? But I feel it is important to raise these awkward and unlikely topics. The more a patient is comfortable with how you come across and the more they buy into what you are trying to achieve for them, the more cooperative they will naturally be.

Training in bedside manners has come a long way, even in my time. Hospital consultants were not altogether well regarded when I was growing up. Like that caricature of a hospital surgeon, Sir Lancelot Spratt, from the *Doctor* novels and films, a consultant was seen as one who took a lot of the credit without doing much of the work, flitting around the hospital wards trailed by teams of nurses, young doctors and medical students, pronouncing on the health, or otherwise, of the poor patients. He was the epitome of arrogance, more interested in having his own ego massaged than doing what was best for his patients. Like many others of my and the previous generation, I grew up believing that consultants were swaggering monsters with a God complex.

Indeed, when we did ward rounds as students, there was still an element of this – as, of course, there still can be, depending on the personalities involved – and it seemed at times that patients were there for the consultants and senior registrars to make us look like the medical idiots we were then. When I eventually got to be a consultant I still would (and sometimes still do) give the students I feel are underperforming a hard time, but the patient is no longer a peripheral figure to be used for teaching purposes. We will have introduced ourselves properly and the patient will know, I hope, that we are all doing our best for them as a person.

Every day we do a pre-ward-round review of all of the patients under our care to ensure we have the details of any recent test results correct, and to discuss how we think we can make each patient better as quickly and safely as possible. We discuss any sensitive issues that might arise, and how best to tell patients and their families any bad news. Once we are clear on each of our roles, we will visit with each patient at their bedside, and I will introduce myself and shake their hands to wish them good morning.

So, though we do our utmost to ensure that patients don't feel like teaching tools, we do still have to teach the medical students by the bedside when we can. Almost all patients kindly agree to this, though everyone understands when they don't. Many patients say they love getting involved in the teaching, and tell me afterwards that, while listening to me explaining their medical issues to students, they learn a lot themselves. I always take note of this, because it means that, contrary to my best efforts, if some are getting more from me in 'teaching mode' rather than 'doctor mode', I need to do better on the communications front. I try to introduce each team member to the patients, so they know exactly who is listening to their personal information. (Strict confidentiality is a given, of course, but if a student comes across someone they know – say, a neighbour from home – they may opt out of the session.) If I ask a student to examine the patient – check a reflex, for example – I ask that they introduce themselves and explain what they have been asked to do in plain English, rather than in medical jargon.

Looking back at my own early days, one of the great joys of being a young doctor was feeling a new-found sense of responsibility. By being in hospital for so many hours on each shift, we got to know our patients intimately. We felt a bit like 'inmates' ourselves, and would see close-up the subtle changes that would occur throughout the day in a hospital. Walking the wards late at night you became more aware of the noises that might keep you awake if you were a patient – the rattling trolleys, the frantic cardiac arrest calls, someone humming a tune as they walked along a corridor. Ireland is such a small country, and almost-without-fail long weekends on call in hospitals as a junior doctor brought this home to me; when chatting to patients and relatives you would make some connection between your family and friends and theirs.

I recall delightful conversations with the elderly patients in my first job on a geriatric ward. They would tell their stories, not just as lists of medical problems to be solved, but as part of the arc of their lives as a whole. Hearing about their upbringings in a different era, and learning first-hand how unbelievably poor many Irish people were for so long, was a lesson in social history and quite an eye-opening experience. The patients brought the story of the country alive for me and I learned more from them than I had done in years of schooling. They seemed to revel in their tales of woe, but would do so with a smile. The late-night chats and realizing how much you were helping them was immensely satisfying. And they understood how young and green we were as doctors and made excuses on our behalf to the senior medics or surgeons when we couldn't find their x-rays or forgot their blood results.

As medical students and junior doctors we had a deep sense of camaraderie – that we were all in it together. We would go in on Saturday morning and not leave the hospital until Monday evening. After twenty-four hours we were paid half time and after forty-eight hours we were not paid at all. This is inconceivable to the junior doctors of today and, with the introduction of the European Working Time directive that limits the hours doctors are legally allowed to work, the team structure we were weaned on has become fractured. Less ridiculous hours is, of course, a good and humane thing, but I wonder if the loss of a sense of belonging has led to a sense of isolation for some of our young trainees.

We all have our good days and our bad days at work, but a bad day as a young doctor might involve watching someone in terrible pain or seeing multiple people die. It is a terribly difficult burden to bear alone and, when you finish your shorter shift after one such bad day and return to your flat to sleep, dark thoughts about your future in medicine must be difficult to deal with. When we had such bad days as young doctors, we rarely left the hospital but instead shared our tales of woe through chats in the doctors' mess – often with older doctors who had been there, done that and lived to tell the tales, who were there to remind us that all was not so bleak. While young doctors' hours and pay are better these days, the expectations of them emotionally are the same. Perhaps this is why many of them appear to feel somewhat disgruntled and unsupported.

Most medical students start their careers with deep empathy for their patients, beginning with their diagnosis and down the sometimes long road of treatment, but in time a protective shell of cynicism can creep in. The long hours and late nights are very draining. The nonsensical calls to chart paracetamol in the middle of the night can harden a young doctor's attitude. Couple this with the daily encounters with the depredations of disease and death and one has to develop a sense of detachment or risk becoming a complete wreck. (I travelled this road myself – I found myself a little cynical after a few years as a young doctor – but with a combination of experience and people close to me getting older, developing illnesses and relating their experiences, both good and bad, with doctors, my sense of empathy has been renewed.)

I only left home to live with friends when I got paid after my first month as an intern. I was twenty-three years old. In my first few years as a doctor, I earned less than a thousand pounds a month while working anywhere from seventy to 100 hours each week. We lived in a world where career progress was slow and the money relatively meagre compared to the work you put in. Yet we were having the time of our lives and felt indestructible – we would manage to go to the nurses' parties in the Mont Clare Hotel on a Monday night on a few hours' sleep, having been in work since Saturday morning. I still had to study for yet more exams, and eventually got my Membership of the Royal College of Physicians, which meant I could go to the next stage of my career and start to train as a neurologist. I was twenty-six years old and started to move from hospital to hospital in Dublin. Every six months or so I would take up a new post, meet new friends and colleagues and learn about how each hospital worked. By the time I had got to know each new system I would have to move on again, an aspect of medical life that has not changed much for young doctors today. It may seem very unsettling but I found it tremendously exciting.

At twenty-eight I was in London, working as a junior registrar. I recall walking home with a takeaway McDonald's one evening when a flash car beeped at me. The car pulled over and out popped an old schoolmate from Dublin. I remember how self-conscious I felt, hiding the McDonald's bag beneath my coat as he regaled me with tales of the buckets of money he was making in 'the City'. I shouldn't have cared, but I did. I was hardly on skid row, but he had bought a house and car, and, most important to me, seemed so much more grown up than I was, as I headed back to my shared flat in Lilley Road with my cold Big Mac. I was bemused that ten years after we had left school I was working ridiculous hours, albeit in a job I loved, but with little or nothing tangible to show for it. Yet, even as a junior doctor, I felt I was needed. I had a purpose that money could not buy.

27
THE PRICE OF SAYING 'YES'
TO THE DRESS

Janine had not been sleeping well. She would wake in her West London flat at 3, 4 and 5 a.m., as if an alarm clock was going off on the hour. Her recurring dream was of a small elephant walking slowly in front of her family and friends, a forlorn look on their faces, as the sounds of a Durban school band echoed in her ears.

Her wedding was in three months' time and she was worried. Not about her decision to get married – Giles was definitely The One. Nor was she concerned about having the ceremony in her native South Africa, the ongoing long-distance rows with the wedding planner notwithstanding. What was really causing her sleeplessness was the fact that she was three stone heavier now than when she and Giles had met two years earlier. Domino's pizzas and nightly video rentals had turned her into what she referred to as 'the blob'. She had been so sure she would lose weight she had persuaded the bridal shop to order a dress two sizes smaller than she then was. They told her that of course she would lose the weight; every bride did. Now they were making noises about letting out the seams and sewing in extra panels.

She had tried various diets, each one more extreme than the last. Her net weight loss: a miserly four pounds. In desperation she joined a local gym and signed up with a prohibitively expensive personal trainer. Finally, the weight started to shift. She ate hardly anything, walked to work instead of taking the Tube, and gave up alcohol. Life was miserable but at least she was getting thinner. Four weeks into this desperation regime and she had shed a stone. She decided to up her game by taking laxatives. In two weeks she had lost another half-stone. She felt tired and wretched, but at least everyone was telling her she looked great and it looked like she'd get into her wedding dress after all.

On her way to her next punishing gym session, she tripped over her gym bag as she tried to haul it out of the car. Both of her legs suddenly felt numb and, as she made her way inside, she tripped again, this time falling flat on to the tarmac. She picked herself up hurriedly, took two further steps and realized that her feet were not doing what they should. To propel herself forward she had to lift her legs high off the ground. Her walk reminded her of the images of astronauts walking on the moon; she knew that if she did not imitate their high-stepping movements her feet would remain stuck to the earth and she would go over once again.

Janine came to visit the Central London hospital where I was working about six weeks before the big day. The loud slapping of her feet on the hospital linoleum made the diagnosis more acoustic than visual. She just could not lift her feet off the ground. When she walked it was with great effort from her upper thigh muscles. The noisy slapping of her feet accentuated her embarrassment and prompted a torrent of anxious tears.

Although it was clear she had foot drop, I did not know why and thus could not adequately comfort her. It did not take long to explain how this had happened – she had damaged both of the nerves that controlled her ability to lift her feet off the ground. It took longer, however, to find out why. I asked the usual questions about changes in medication, family history and whether she had had any previous medical problems, but to no avail. It was the trip over the gym bag that was key. And so I got the whole story of her mad bid to lose over two stone in three months.

As a result of dieting and exercising like a woman possessed Janine had lost the fat protecting the nerves near her knee joints so they had been inadvertently exposed. These nerves run down to our feet and control dorsiflexion of the foot – the movement we produce when we walk on our heels. Being more exposed, the nerves were easily compressed; for example, by crossing her legs when sitting at meetings at work. Eventually, the nerves controlling the muscles of her ankles and feet were damaged to the point where they could no longer transmit the electric current required and ceased working altogether, leading to Janine's pre-nuptial 'dropped' feet. It is a common problem in people who lose weight precipitously either by design or through illness. It is a fairly common sight in patients with cancer or in some who have spent prolonged periods in intensive care.

The nerves would recover slowly over the next month or two, and Janine's fears of a wheelchair-bound future were put to rest. But the wedding had to be postponed. I later learned that she recovered full function of her legs and went on to marry Giles later that year. She walked up the aisle the same size she was before the nightmares of elephants had started.

Younger doctors, who lack experience in medicine and in life, can sometimes seize upon the vices of their patients to chastise them. Contrary to their deserved reputation for prolific drinking, young doctors may seem very mean, lecturing already anxious patients many years their seniors. Over time I realized this was a small defence mechanism to manage their own (my own, in my early years) ignorance. After all, it is easier to blame a patient for their illness, and thus exacerbate their shame and misery, than think through the problem in depth and admit how little you actually know.

Silvia was fifty-six years old, right-handed and originally from Croatia. The pressure of a late-in-life course to become a reiki instructor was getting her down. Her two children had left home a few years previously. The 'Is that it?' of the empty nester was a cliché she tried to stave off by devoting herself to her studies, but it wasn't helping. She was drinking more than she used to, but denied it was a crutch until she woke up in a blur one Monday afternoon and was unable to move her right arm.

She tried to convince herself that she had had a stroke, as this was far more palatable to her than having to face the truth of her descent into alcohol dependence. Her wine o'clock drinking had escalated to gin and tonics for lunch, and things deteriorated from there. She had downed a half-litre of Hendricks on her own that Monday while watching daytime television instead of writing up her assignment.

Silvia had already searched for possible causes for her weak arm on the internet and quickly came up with 'Saturday night palsy'. This pejorative phrase was coined by doctors many years ago for drunks who fall asleep with their arms draped over the back of a chair, compressing the radial nerve in the spiral groove of the humerus. It results in a 'dropped wrist' (like Janine's dropped foot) and usually recovers within four to six weeks – although the sense of shame probably lasts a lot longer than the hangover. (In fact, the term is thought to have been used to describe wrist drop in young men courting on park benches in more chaste times in London, a much more romantic image but, I imagine, rather difficult to explain to partners if the romances were of an illicit nature.)

Silvia was initially reluctant to engage with me, but softened when she realized she was not being judged. I was able to agree with her own diagnosis, which made her feel better – not only was it a temporary state of affairs but she had managed to do a sensible bit of research about it too. I didn't have to say anything about her drinking because she knew well herself that she had had a wake-up call. Silvia's arm recovered within a few days and, of course, she swore off alcohol for ever.

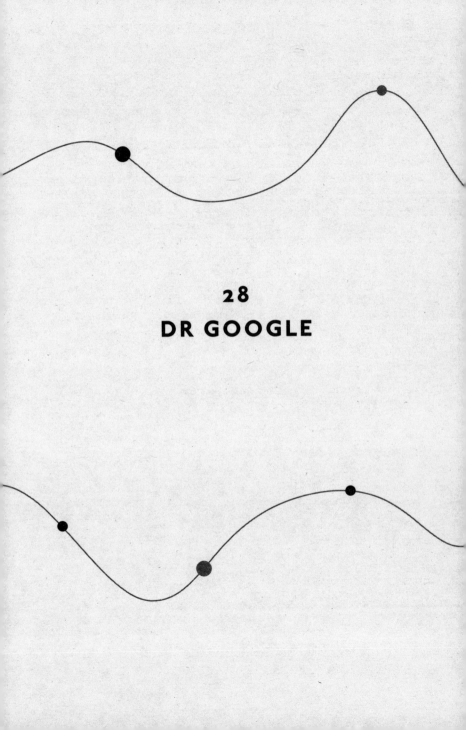

28
DR GOOGLE

My first job as a schoolboy was picking strawberries with friends. We were paid two pence for each punnet and, to a ten-year-old boy, this was a fortune. I was always a fairly competitive soul with a decent work ethic so I would arrive early each summer's day to the local strawberry field owned by the parish priests in our area, and try and out-pick my friends. After hours of kneeling in the dry soil I would stand to find one or other of my feet was numb. Sometimes it would be more severe and for a brief few moments my foot would be weak (dropped foot – there it is again). I would massage the leg and run it off before getting back to competitive strawberry picking.

I would later discover that 'strawberry picker's foot drop' was a well-described phenomenon in neurology. Being a skinny fellow, this transient foot drop could occur over the subsequent years whenever I even sat with my legs crossed for prolonged periods. Like most people, from time to time I would also wake up with a numb hand having slept in an awkward position. I would shake my numb hand briskly, leading to return of full feeling, and get on with my day.

As I began to learn about all things neurological, I started to understand the mechanics of nerve compression. What, to me, was a simple transient compression of the median or ulnar nerves to my hands, I soon became aware represented the first signs of multiple sclerosis or motor neuron disease to those who were not as fortunate and who had turned to Dr Google for enlightenment.

Professor Jean-Martin Charcot is regarded as the father of modern neurology. He worked in the famous Pitié-Salpêtrière Hospital in Paris in the late nineteenth century. (I was fortunate enough to spend almost a year there during my training. I did not speak much French but the people there could not have been more welcoming, and I immersed myself in the history of the subject that I love.) Charcot was a brilliant clinician and teacher and took a particular interest in what he called hysterical behaviour. At public lectures he would demonstrate what was known at that time about all things neurological and bring in subjects whom he felt were feigning their illnesses (of course, these being sexist times, they were nearly always women). Charcot is believed to have spoken, over 130 years ago, about 'la maladie du petit papier' (roughly translated as 'disease of the small piece of paper'). Patients would arrive at the clinic with scraps of paper on which they detailed all of their symptoms. The longer the list, the less likely he felt that he was dealing with a serious neurological illness. Sir William Osler, another giant of medical history, known as one of the fathers of modern medicine, termed the condition 'neurasthenia'.

Far from labelling it 'la maladie du petit papier', I think the use of lists and diaries detailing neurological illnesses can be extremely helpful. I encourage patients to write down their symptoms, the timelines, any variations, and things that provoke or alleviate these symptoms. I believe it helps people to focus on what they truly want out of a consultation. And it can give them back a much-needed sense of control. For someone with migraine, for example, tracking what makes their headaches better or worse makes the patient an active participant in figuring out a treatment plan.

However, like most things in life, problems arise when the behaviour is taken to extremes. We are now in the age, as it has been called elsewhere, of 'la maladie du grand printout'. Today we have not just plain lists but pages of printed-out notes, spreadsheets of symptoms and even timelines stretching back decades – all to be covered in a thirty-minute consultation while the queues of patients build up outside.

Extensive Google searches will yield multiple possible diagnoses and, human nature being as it is, we will invariably latch on to the worst-case scenario that fits with our symptoms. As often as not, the doctor is forced to exclude the patient's diagnosis and, when they do, the disbelieving patient may go elsewhere and the process begins all over again.

One of my rules in the internet age is to tell young doctors never to trust the findings of someone who comes with a Google diagnosis, and never to trust anyone who says they have not googled their symptoms. We all do it, neurologists included, so we might as well at least start the conversation as honestly as we can.

Imelda was eighty-five and accompanied by her three grown children, who had spent the summer months watching their mother list drunkenly around the house, dizzy spells interspersed with episodic vomiting, and then she would take to her bed. Imelda looked great and had a fine sense of humour, but had lost her self-confidence. This can happen with people who are lucky enough to have been pretty healthy well into old age and finally experience ill-health.

Her previous scans were all clear, her children assured me, but they had done their research, and each had come to their own conclusion. Her son was sure she had Parkinson's; her two daughters thought that she was having recurrent strokes. Imelda sat there petrified as they made their diagnostic pronouncements.

Imelda told me that she had been having dizzy spells for well over thirty years. As usual, I wanted her to recall when this had first happened. It was striking how, with only the slightest prompting, she was able to do this. Imelda had gone on holiday to Italy with four friends around the time of her fiftieth birthday. She had been very excited about it, and looked forward to the trip away with 'the girls' for months. She felt she had overdone the wine on the first night and wanted to sit by the pool the next day to recover, but as she walked from the lift to the sun loungers she noticed she was listing to the left.

'Oh my God,' she recalled. 'I really had overdone it, and I thought I was still drunk.' Imelda was very lady-like and you could see this was not her form at all. Even thirty-five years later, she blushed just retelling the story.

The dizzy spells settled for a while and she got on with things, but intermittently over the next thirty-five years Imelda would experience these horrendous spells when she would walk 'drunkenly'. She gave up alcohol altogether, just in case it was the cause. She would sometimes be confined to her bed for a week or more, her world turned upside down whenever she moved her head. She felt her head was constantly 'muzzy' for all of those years.

From time to time she had sought help, but only got the occasional period of respite from the medications her GP prescribed. She stood in front of me, and when asked to close her eyes she started to sway as if caught in a strong wind. Her eyes would stutter when she looked from left to right, and she couldn't walk easily in a straight line on the clinic room floor. 'You do think I'm drunk!' she laughed.

Happily, Imelda just had chronic vertigo, due to an imbalance in the fluid of her inner ear, and totally unrelated to her alcohol intake. With a lot of physiotherapy, her balance problems could at least be significantly improved and possibly cured entirely. In this case Dr Google, and Imelda's children, had got it wrong.

Aishling had beautiful red hair, but it had a tendency to curl which was 'not cool', she explained. 'I have been straightening my hair since I was fifteen,' she said, 'and never had any problems until the last few months. Now, I can only straighten one side of my hair and then my arms are too tired to finish the job, so unless Mum helps me I am left with one side straight and the other side curly and my brother now calls me "Sideshow Bob" [a character from *The Simpsons*].'

As my long-haired registrar stifled her mirth at my ignorance, Aishling produced her GHD. Given my follicularly challenged state she had to explain what it was. GHD stands for 'Good Hair Day' and it is the brand name of one of the bestselling electrical hair straighteners. It looks like a pair of tongs, but when plugged in it heats up to become a clamping iron in which the long hair is gripped and slowly straightened. To straighten Aishling's luxuriant locks took about twenty minutes on each side.

The neurological examination of Aishling's arms was normal. She had good power, no loss of muscle bulk, and all her arm reflexes were present. When she held her arms up above her head for a few minutes they appeared to go a shade paler. I took her pulse in both arms with her arms down by her sides and then with her hands held above her head. After a minute or so the strength of the pulse to both hands diminished appreciably and Aishling reported that her arms were too tired to hold up any longer. It was clear that something was interrupting the blood flow to her hands but only when they were held above shoulder level for a few minutes.

An x-ray of Aishling's neck revealed an extra rib in the neck area, known as a cervical rib, that would have been there from birth. Sometimes fibrous bands associated with the extra rib can compress the blood vessels coming from the heart to the arms and so the symptoms would come on only when her arms were raised above her head. A relatively simple surgical procedure cuts these bands and relieves the pressure on the circulatory defect. Aishling underwent such a procedure and was soon back to her good hair days.

Within three weeks of seeing Aishling I met Siobhán. She was twenty-two years old and complained of pain in her arms for the previous year.

'Do you have a GHD?' I asked.

'How did you know?' she replied with a quizzical smile. 'I got a GHD for Christmas last year but over the last few months I have been unable to use it, as my arms get tired when I am using it before a night out – it's ruining my social life!'

It is not uncommon to see a case such as Aishling's, hear about GHDs and the like for the first time, and then, like buses, see similar cases in quick succession. I am sure there is a certain bias in this non-scientific method and, of course, I always fear I have missed many such cases before by not being alert enough to ask the right questions.

I went through the same examination with Siobhán as I had with Aishling. Once again the strength of her pulse diminished rapidly when I held her arms above her head for a few minutes. Feeling smug, I ordered the x-ray to confirm the cervical ribs and was deflated when they confirmed nothing of the kind. I requested an MRI scan of her neck and of the forest of nerves around the armpit regions, and here we found a narrowing of the blood vessels to her arms.

With some further blood tests and scans we were able to determine that Siobhán had a rare inflammation of the blood vessels throughout her body, though only those to her arms were causing any symptoms, but intermittently and particularly when using her hair straightener.

With medications to reduce the inflammation she was eventually back to herself and her straight hair, although by now she had grown used to her 'new look' and abandoned the GHD anyway.

Both of these young women had similar symptoms and similar signs on examination and both blamed their GHD. Yet the cause for each was very different, and for Siobhán it meant heavy-duty medication for over two years to alleviate her pain. These are good examples, I think, when trying to illustrate how self-diagnosis via Google can be unreliable. Many conditions can match someone's complaints and cause either panic ('Oh my God, I have a vasculitis and will need steroids for ever') or undue reassurance ('Ah sure, it is only a little extra rib').

One of the great secrets of modern medicine is that doctors are training to treat the sick but are in fact frequently treating the well. It is fairly basic pop psychology to understand the worried well. People with headaches brought on by the stresses of their jobs are convinced they have a brain tumour. Our minds are so cluttered we cannot store all of the information we are exposed to, so inevitably we start to forget things and then worry that we are developing dementia. The hand that is numb in the morning because we slept awkwardly provokes concerns about MS. And, again, Dr Google is not always the friend of the worried well.

Raising awareness of chronic illness is a goal of many charitable organizations. I greatly admire their endeavours, as the people who suffer from as yet incurable illnesses appear to regain a sense of control when they get involved in such drives to raise awareness, and millions of euros are raised to help researchers better understand difficult conditions and work towards an eventual cure.

The Ice Bucket challenge was devised by someone with an iPhone and an interest in raising money for motor neuron disease and was performed as a wheeze. It raised millions, and fast, and was quickly seen as the go-to route to raise money for relatively rare illnesses.

What happened next was unprecedented though. What became apparent in my clinics – and I presume those of other neurologists – was that awareness, now raised, had led to hyper-awareness and, in many cases, to borderline hypochondriasis. Around the time of 'the Challenge', I encountered numerous young men at their wits' end asking whether they were dying of this terrible disease. It was difficult to reassure them on clinical or statistical grounds. And when all of the tests proved normal or negative, I would hear from neurology colleagues that they had been asked for second or third opinions.

At the root of their anxieties the social history appeared critical – middle-class (usually) white males who had recently become fathers for the first time. The men were worried that they would not be around to see their newborns grow to adulthood.

This cannot be the only generation of young fathers who have experienced such angst, but this highly specific manifestation of their worries in the wake of a social-media-led awareness campaign was new to me. I did not diagnose a single case of motor neuron disease among this worried group. But I wonder if they ever recovered their full peace of mind.

Likewise, for many years I have seen young mothers present with numb hands or feet or pins and needles in their extremities, and they are generally worried about multiple sclerosis. It seems particular to young Irish mothers who are aware that they are in the most frequent demographic category affected by MS – young, white and female. All they can see ahead is a future with wheelchairs.

While occasionally I have diagnosed MS, most of the women who presented have turned out not to have it. It is curious to me that men seem to worry more about developing motor neuron disease and women about developing MS, but both groups seem, at heart, to be worried about not being there for their children. Giving patients the 'all clear' is one of the great joys of my working life. After all, it is pretty easy, as a doctor, to look after those who are well.

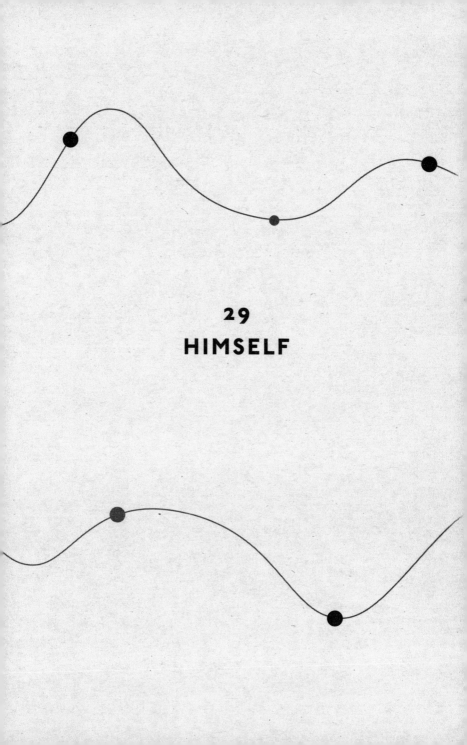

29
HIMSELF

After leaving Ireland in 1995 I spent many happy years in various hospitals throughout central London before moving to Paris for a year and to Melbourne in 2000. I had brilliant fun as a peripatetic neurologist, but I missed Ireland and was keen to get home. And that's why, almost ten years after leaving Dublin, I found myself sitting in front of what seemed to me like a huge panel of senior colleagues in St Vincent's Hospital feeling like an eighteen-year-old first-year medical student once more, being interviewed for a consultant-neurologist post.

I worked very hard at my interview preparation as there were at least ten other suitable (possibly more suitable) candidates for the job, so there was much excitement among the small but loosely knit community of Dublin neurology. This was to be only the twelfth or thirteenth consultant neurologist appointed in Ireland at that time.

I remember the ill-fitting suit I wore and the nervous attempts at raising a smile from the forbidding panel of my future peers – how not to do an interview, according to all of the advice I have read on the subject since. That evening I was catching up with friends with whom I had shared many of the ups and downs of medical student life, expressing resignation about how badly it had gone and anticipating the long flight back to Melbourne, when I got the call offering me the post. Quite overwhelmed and very much out of character, I shed a tear. I was ecstatic. I guess my somewhat naïve authenticity had somehow won the day.

Having packed my life up once again, and said goodbye to Australia, I was very excited to arrive in St Vincent's some months later. While I felt ready for it, I was still extremely nervous. My senior colleague Michael (known to one and all as 'Hutch') had worked single-handedly as the hospital neurologist for over twenty years and appeared pleased to finally have a colleague, albeit a much younger and greener one. The relationship between colleagues in medicine is described as more difficult than a marriage as you can always divorce your spouse but you are stuck with colleagues – and they with you – for life.

When I arrived Hutch said, 'Great, you're here at last, you can take over!'

He was joking – but he promptly left the ward and I like to think he went out that evening and got gently drunk with relief after all of the years he had carried neurology in the hospital on his own.

One of my first tasks, and one that will remain with me for ever, was to explain to a family of six adult children that their mother, who was in the end stages of motor neuron disease, was dying. It was impossible to be precise about when, but I was qualified thirteen years by this stage, and experience told me that she had no more than a few months to live.

I explained the eighty-year-old woman's circumstances confidently – and, I hope, sympathetically – to her children, who ranged in age, I estimated, between about forty and fifty-five. They knew she would soon be dead, and had come to terms with it as best they could, but were keen to have greater clarity as to when and how the end would come. I told them that I believed she had between three and six months to live, with the usual caveats of 'it could be less, it could be more', and that we would do all we could to avoid her suffering any further.

I often wonder what goes through the minds of patients and family when a relatively fresh-faced doctor explains a sad case like this. You can see them glazing over as you explain the more complex medical details, but you assume they will remember for ever some of the words you use. Indeed, this family was probably going to remember even the peeling wallpaper in the 'relatives' rooms' we then used for breaking such sad news.

I finished my monologue and asked whether they had any questions. After a brief silence, the eldest son piped up. 'Well, Doctor, how long has she got?' I was disappointed with myself that, in spite of my best efforts, I had obviously not been clear.

'About three to six months,' I repeated. 'It could be more, it could be less.'

He received this seemingly new information with a grim but accepting shake of his head.

The room once again went silent and I edged forward in my seat before asking, 'Does anyone else have any questions?'

His sister spoke next. 'I want to know, Doctor, how long you think she has?'

I got slightly flustered. Here was my first task on my first day, and

I was falling at the first hurdle. I appreciated the intense nature of the conversation. I had done this many times before while working abroad: this grieving family was not taking in a word I was saying.

'Three to six months; could be more, could be less. One can never be sure about these things. I am really sorry you are all going through this awful ordeal.'

I waited. Silence again. Had the terrible news finally begun to sink in . . . perhaps?

I thanked them for listening – what else could I say? – and got up to give them some privacy for a while. I said I would come back later in case they had any further questions. As I reached for the door handle, the youngest of the six siblings let out a yelp.

'I have just one more question!'

I was dumbfounded. I spun around and started to repeat myself.

'About three to six months; could be more, could be less –'

'No, it's a different question,' she cut across me. I was relieved, if a little embarrassed at my display of exasperation.

'Are you anything to Himself?'

The trials of having a famous brother had begun.

What had never occurred to me when returning to Ireland was that having a brother who worked in television would have any impact on me. Of course, during my long sojourn abroad Ryan's career had developed, but before coming home I had no idea how high his profile was. I was soon to learn.

A decade later and an oncology colleague asked me to look at one of her patients. Mrs O'Reilly was about sixty-two years old and had been well until a few months previously. A niggling but persistent pain in her right flank eventually persuaded her to see her GP. Within a few weeks she was undergoing her first round of chemotherapy. The chemotherapy was not working and she had developed a weak right hand.

I walked into her room. Her distraught husband was sitting beside this frail lady who now looked many years older than him. I thought he was her son initially. The brief few months of her illness and her treatment had aged the poor woman terribly. Her emaciated frame was topped with her beanie hat ('the new bandana', her daughter told me with a smile). I introduced myself and explained why I had been asked to see her – to investigate her weak right hand.

Her left eye was closed and, when I asked her why, she casually mentioned some double vision for the previous few weeks that she attributed to an allergy to some new eye make-up.

As we chatted she started to giggle. It was undoubtedly a pleasant interaction but the humour in it eluded me. From the neurological perspective she had a third-nerve palsy (paralysis of one of the nerves to the muscles that move your eyeballs and keep your eyelids open) of her left eye, no feeling on the left side of her face and a decidedly weak and clumsy right arm and leg.

Her quiet giggling continued as, apologetically, I scratched her feet to elicit the plantar response. Her right big toe went up (a bad sign) and she laughed again. As I started to tell her that I was concerned, but not absolutely sure yet, that her cancer might have spread to her brain, she interrupted me.

'I feel like I am meeting Himself.'

By now, after years of getting a similar response to my apparent resemblance – in manner and voice, if not appearance – to my younger brother, I was well used to this happening. Having had a long and intense conversation with a patient about a life-changing, or even life-ending, diagnosis, I usually finish by asking if the patient has any further questions. Frequently there is a question about Ryan, or a joke about getting tickets for his show. It took me quite a while to stop being surprised at how many times a week this would happen. It was comedy of the blackest nature. As I got older I realized that my sense of disbelief was in poor spirit. If it was a distraction for people at a difficult moment what harm was it doing? As I keep reminding myself – 'Whatever works.'

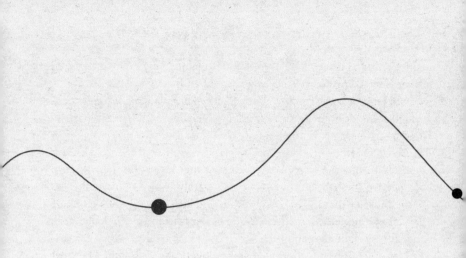

30
A SHAKING PALSY

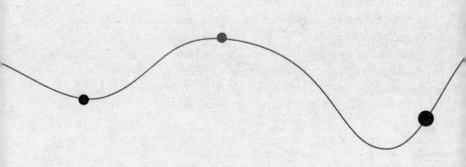

Conor was writing a cheque in the bank and the queue was building behind him. He could feel the Friday afternoon crowd's impatience when he dropped his chequebook on the floor and fumbled as he tried to pick it up. He felt sweat trickling down his back and his face start to burn. The bank clerk smiled and asked him to sign on the line. He paused. He couldn't do it. He reddened further and asked her to take the cheque unsigned but she said she couldn't. He tried again. The pen felt like a lead weight in his shaking hand. He tried to scrawl his signature but the result was unrecognizable. His usually neat handwriting was indecipherable. He could hardly read the tiny, spidery writing himself. The bank clerk reluctantly accepted the cheque. Conor hurried out of the bank past the glaring customers. 'They thought I was drunk, I'm sure,' he told me later. He felt both humiliated and frightened, and his embarrassment finally convinced him to seek help.

He was sixty-three and had worked in marketing for years. He was happily married and financially comfortable. His children were grown up and he was a proud grandfather twice over. Friday nights were spent with his old school mates, and he had a season ticket for the Leinster rugby matches. On the face of it, life was pretty good.

But Conor had known something was wrong for about a year. Everything had felt terribly non-specific, but anxiety was creeping into every part of his life. He realized that he was increasingly hampered buttoning his shirt for work in the mornings. Then in the office he felt he was constantly rushing, though he was clearly slowing down. He noted that his colleagues would walk ahead of him when heading out for lunch and it was tiring for him to keep up with them. He sighed at what he thought were the vicissitudes of age.

Now and again, when he was watching television, his right hand would tremble a little, and he would hide it from Gráinne. He hadn't shared his worries with her, but he was tossing and turning a lot at night and she complained about him kicking her in his sleep. He put it down to nightmares. So now she was sleeping badly, too.

He did not feel old but he began to think that the man looking back at him in the mirror was ageing rapidly. His granddaughter started to imitate him one Sunday as they walked Dun Laoghaire pier. She mimicked a hunched-over old man. He laughed, but was secretly horrified. 'Is this how she sees me? Is this how she'll remember me when I'm gone?'

Retirement loomed and he fretted from time to time about what he would do with his days. He loved his job and didn't want to retire, so, he reasoned, the worry was probably distracting him as he got ready in the morning. He laughed at the irony of all the young people who complained about stress at work; here he was, heading into retirement, stressing about not working.

Try as he might to ignore the gathering storm, it was the little things that slowly but surely broke his self-confidence. He held the bannister of the stairs more firmly. He took the lift at work when previously he would have bounded up the stairs. The shake in his right hand became more persistent, and eventually he began to eat lunch alone, telling colleagues he had too much to do and couldn't go out for the usual soup and sandwiches. He knew full well he couldn't manage soup, as the spoon had started to sway on its way to his lips. He isolated himself for fear of being found out, though he didn't know what he was trying to hide.

Gráinne had noticed the change in Conor's walk, and felt awful nagging him to stand up straight when she saw him turning into an old man before her eyes. She had also noticed that during their evening walks by the sea Conor seemed to swing one arm and hold his right arm rigidly by his side. 'It reminded me of the scene in *Catch 22*, when the troops took to walking with their arms straight down,' she said later.

Yet she joined in the lie that the changes were due to her husband's anxiety about his imminent retirement. She was nervous about the retirement herself – what would all that time together do to their relationship? She hadn't gone out to work since they'd married over thirty years earlier, and since the kids had left home, she had settled in to the slower pace of her life without them. She was used to having the house to herself each day.

Their eldest daughter got engaged and they held a party in the family home. People reflect on their lives and relationships at times like this; it's a time to see everyone together, observe how things have changed since the last big celebration. As Gráinne looked fondly on her family celebrating this latest good news, she caught a glimpse of Conor, unsmiling in the corner and avoiding the throng while pretending to busy himself mixing drinks. This wasn't like him at all. She was used to gently upbraiding her husband for his excesses and 'any excuse for a party' attitude. Thank God she hadn't married a boring man, she had always thought.

At breakfast the next morning, they spoke about the night before. Conor seemed distracted, and she teased him for being hungover and mumbling. As he buttered the breakfast toast she saw his right hand shaking. She knew in her heart where this was going.

For a while, she avoided Google for fear of what she might find, but after a few weeks she couldn't hold back any longer. By the time she had finished searching, she was in tears. She had typed in 'tremor' and got Parkinson's disease, as she had expected, but as she was led from one website to another she spiralled into a neurological nightmare of brain cancer and motor neuron disease.

'Oh my God, Conor is going to die. Or worse, he'll have to live as a vegetable,' she thought. She rang their old friend who was also their GP and made an appointment for as soon as she could get one. She had not discussed this with Conor, who continued to work away. So often this happens: two people who have spent their adult lives together have the same fears at the same time but do not share them. It seems both protective and defensive – not wanting to face illness in yourself or your partner, hoping that nothing will change.

When Conor got home to the news he was seeing the family doctor the following morning, they had the first of many arguments about it. He was outraged. He was embarrassed that what he thought was only apparent to himself was just as obvious to everyone else. Gráinne said she was worried about his shaking, and just wanted to make sure he was OK, but he was angry and felt betrayed. So they both spent a sleepless night in separate rooms.

By morning, things had thawed, and they held hands as they waited to see the GP. Conor suddenly felt ancient, and later said he could only see 'all the old people' in the waiting room – and he felt like one of them.

The doctor called them in, and I would guess had made the diagnosis by the time they had sat down. He had gone to rugby matches with Conor over the years, and many an International weekend was spent in Dublin or 'on tour' on the Continent, drinking a bit more than was good for them perhaps, but always having a great time. In front of him sat his good friend, who was only a few years younger than him, but who looked like he'd aged ten years since the last rugby season. He told them he couldn't be absolutely sure, but suspected that Conor had Parkinson's disease. Their world crumbled when they heard the actual words – even though they would later admit that this was exactly what they had suspected.

A few weeks later, Conor and his wife came to see me. My secretary came into the office to tell me he was here and, sotto voce, said, 'I think he has Parkinson's.' We had been working together for some time, and despite her young age she was well able to distinguish the worried well from the truly unwell.

'Why do you think so?' I asked.

'He looks like one of those Hollywood stars who's had too much Botox, and he walks like he's seventy-five. His referral letter says he's sixty-three.'

I brought them in and as they sat down in the office I could feel the fear – theirs and, to a lesser degree, mine. Knowing that their GP had already brought up Parkinson's, I asked whether they had been googling; he said no, but she quietly said, 'Just a little bit.' He scowled at her; it was plainly news to him.

I describe Parkinson's to patients as like a car running out of petrol, but the fuel in this case is dopamine, a neurotransmitter responsible for conveying information to specific nerve cells from the brain. We start out life with a full tank of dopamine, but for most of us, as we age, our reserves are running out. At some stage, people who develop symptoms of Parkinson's have reached a critically low level of their natural dopamine.

While Conor's diagnosis was as immediately evident to me as it had been to their GP and our secretary, I had to be careful to make sure that I was not missing any other possibilities. Most people with typical symptoms of Parkinson's disease – a hand tremor present when at rest that goes away temporarily when they move; bent posture; reduced swinging of one arm; an expressionless face – have what we call idiopathic or 'regular' Parkinson's disease. This type usually responds well to therapy, at least in the early stages, and often for many years.

There is a much smaller group of people who have what is called 'Parkinson's plus' or 'Parkinson's "extra"', who respond less well to treatment, and the outlook is much more gloomy, hence the 'plus'. These conditions or syndromes look like Parkinson's, bar a few subtle differences, found with a carefully elicited history and a detailed neurological examination. So some poor folk go to the neurologist fearing the worst – Parkinson's – only to find out it's not the worst at all.

Conor and I walked around the room together. Doing this in an examination where Parkinson's is likely allows us, and the patient's watching relatives, to see any differences in posture, arm movements and the ability to turn quickly. Conor shuffled, but speedily, as if he were chasing something, or fearful he might topple over if he lost momentum, like a child learning to ride a bicycle. While most of us have a very fine tremor, if we look closely, when we hold our hands out straight in front of us, Conor had a very visible coarse tremor of his right hand at rest. He smiled briefly when his hand stopped shaking when he held it in a different position, but it soon started up again. When I lifted his right arm up and down it revealed the characteristic stiffness of Parkinson's; it was like trying to bend a lead pipe.

I asked Conor to tap his left foot on the ground as if he were listening to a familiar song. I turned away, the better to listen to the rhythm, and it sounded fine. When he tried the same trick with his right foot, however, it was as if his body had lost all sense of rhythm and the jerky tapping quickly dissipated into a barely audible slap of his foot on the ground. The difference was striking. This relative slowness of movement in one side of the body compared to the other is termed 'bradykinesia' and is a classic symptom, generally more or less diagnostic of Parkinson's disease. Poor Conor could see and hear for himself the disease that he had been trying to cover up for so long.

Conor's eyes twinkled throughout our meeting. His face looked like he was trying to smile, but his expression was frozen. Gráinne sat by stoically. Now and again a tear would run down her face as she watched the whole process from across the room.

Conor had all of the signs of 'regular' Parkinson's disease and there was no evidence of anything 'extra'. Some small solace for me, but not for him at that stage. He and Gráinne reacted calmly to the news that he had an early and, as yet, mild, form of Parkinson's disease. In a sense there was some element of relief, especially for Gráinne, whose research online had uncovered far worse potential diagnoses.

Conor decided there and then that he would retire, saying that he had better get busy living life to the full. I counselled caution; to think carefully about any big decisions over the coming months. I have many patients who have lived with the condition well into their eighties or nineties with relatively few problems; others deteriorate rapidly within a few years of diagnosis, and it is simply impossible to know which road any individual's condition will follow.

I said to Conor that he should take some time to digest the information, have a think about the treatment options, and engage with a physiotherapy class to which I'm accustomed to refer people in a similar situation. In addition, when someone is diagnosed with Parkinson's, it can be incredibly helpful for them to talk to other patients. Being part of a class can lead to a friendly sense of competition, and I've seen patients come back and say, to their delight, that their classmates hardly believe they have the disease sometimes. (Conor took to this healthy sense of one-upmanship with great enthusiasm.) On the other hand, people who can see they are worse off than those around them can often become even more despondent, so we have to be very careful.

When he returned a few weeks later to discuss potential therapies, Conor asked whether he could do without drugs for the moment – he felt great, and thought he didn't need them just yet. I was gratified to see his optimism return, but having suggested he reconsider retiring because the disease might not advance rapidly, I now had to remind him of the flip side: unfortunately, Parkinson's is a progressive condition, so while a patient might feel fine at the moment, or even years from now, it will almost always disimprove.

*

My petrol tank analogy – that Parkinson's is caused when the tank runs low on fuel (the neurotransmitter, dopamine) – though easy to understand as a crude explanation for patients, is faulty. It's not just that the tank is full and then runs out. In truth, a healthy brain commonly produces *more* dopamine than we need – just in case. And, because the human body is at its best a well-balanced system, it also produces enzymes whose job it is to break down the excess of dopamine the brain produces most of our lives. At first, when someone develops Parkinson's symptoms, a neurologist may try to maintain what dopamine their patient still has by giving drugs that stop the enzymes from destroying the extra dopamine the patient now needs. Later, we might use a kind of 'fake' dopamine that stimulates the dopamine receptors – called dopamine agonists – where dopamine usually goes to prevent the disease. Later again, when a patient is struggling – say, to tie their shoe-laces, do up buttons, shave in the morning – we will dispense dopamine itself in tablet form, to be taken throughout the day.

While it's true that there is no cure for Parkinson's disease, the treatments can be very effective. It is the neurologist's job to try and replenish the depleted dopamine with medication. Each drug regimen is specific to each individual, based on when the patient is at their best and their worst every day. This might mean when their tremor is most obvious or when they feel they are at their slowest in terms of their ability to move. We then tailor the amount and frequency of the medication to kick in at the low points (tremors, slowness) and fade away when they briefly feel more like themselves. It gives great hope to the patient and the doctor when they see their facial expressions return, their posture straighten and their tremor abate in the early stages of treatment. This has huge psychological benefit, which can be half the battle for most sufferers. With more optimism, people will willingly engage in physiotherapy. Learning some techniques to manage symptoms boosts the lowered self-esteem a diagnosis can bring. People will start to socialize again, meaning that the brain is stimulated and, crucially, distracted from spiralling gloomy thoughts.

The cliché of the retired golfer has particular poignancy for people with Parkinson's. Many of my patients have looked forward to endless days of trying to lower their handicap once they stop working, but it is on the golf course that they experience their initial symptoms. Difficulty pulling back the putter on the green seems to come first, as they have an issue initiating movements. Many then find it hard to chip the ball, hovering over it with their club, as though lost in thought, but really because they cannot get their brains to engage with their hands to get the ball airborne.

Because golf is such a process-driven game, practised again and again with great attention to detail, it can be a particularly accurate lens through which to measure out a patient's deterioration over time. Golfers cannot fail to face the truth of their decline when they go from playing eighteen holes a day to nine, to needing a golf buggy, to playing the six holes closest to the clubhouse. The perceived social humiliation is painful to hear about, and eventually many give up their hobby, and with it their social outlets, leading to further isolation and melancholy. A vicious cycle then ensues as the psychological fall exacerbates the physical torment.

The longer a person with Parkinson's is on dopamine, the more of it the brain will usually require. The more they need, the more likely it will lead to the development of dyskinesias, or unpredictable writhing movements. It looks like the person is practically dancing all the time whether sitting or standing. It can lead to disfiguring grimacing and, though people who are frozen to a standstill by the condition itself will still get some relief to be moving at all, they and their loved ones can become self-conscious. Simple things, like having a meal in a restaurant, take on enormous significance and I often wonder about the stress the person feels when such public events are arranged. Do they take an extra hit of dopamine before venturing out? If they do, are they worried this will cause their dyskinesia to worsen just as the soup arrives? Many families eventually give up trying to maintain a semblance of their pre-Parkinson's lives, meaning that now it's not only the patient who becomes isolated, but their immediate family as well.

One of my mentors in London was an international expert and a pioneer in the field of Parkinson's for many decades. His advice about the disease has always stayed with me.

'Dr Tubridy,' he exclaimed rather grandly, when I finished presenting the case of a man who had early Parkinson's, 'I have been studying

Parkinson's patients for over thirty years, but what dose of dopamine do *you* think we should give this man?'

I mumbled a few suggestions. In those days, he did his clinics in front of an audience of about twenty visiting students from all over Europe, so it was fairly daunting for the junior doctors, not to mention the patients telling their stories. He smiled at my bumbling efforts.

'Some good suggestions for the average person with Parkinson's, but there is no such thing as "an average person", let alone an average person with Parkinson's disease. After much trial and error, over my many years treating many thousands of people with this condition, I have concluded that the only course of action for a neurologist in this situation is to provide the patient with a bucket of dopamine tablets and instruct them to take them as needed. After a few weeks they will reach an equilibrium, and that is when the neurologist who listens to his patients will know what dose that patient should have.'

His advice to treat each patient as an individual in individual circumstances has stuck with me for over twenty years – though I try to be more parsimonious with the dopamine.

31
TALES OF THE UNEXPECTED

Anne Marie had swum competitively in her younger years and then coached children at her local swimming club, so she had had her fair share of shoulder injuries over the years. These had culminated in an increasing discomfort in her left shoulder when she tried to lift her arms above her head. This is commonly diagnosed as a 'frozen shoulder', and Anne Marie was referred to a physiotherapist. The stiffness eased a little, but after a few months she sought medical help again. An x-ray revealed degenerative changes in the shoulder joint – what medics euphemistically call 'wear and tear' – so she was sent to an orthopaedic surgeon. He injected the shoulder with some steroids, which did alleviate some of her pain, but she still couldn't move her arm freely, particularly when she went for a long run in the morning. The surgeon, having run out of more conservative options, suggested that she might consider shoulder replacement surgery. As she pondered what she considered to be a rather drastic option, she mentioned that she was also now developing an intermittent shake in her left hand. The surgeon said he was not sure what was causing the tremor, and that he felt it was not linked to the shoulder problem. 'I can fix the shoulder, but it probably won't help the shake,' he said.

And that's how Anne Marie ended up in my clinic. She was just fifty-one but had many of the early signs of Parkinson's – she held her left arm stiffly by her side and had the tell-tale resting tremor. She spoke animatedly but in a hoarse whisper. She was married and had two children, but came to the clinic on her own. When I asked about her husband she went quiet. 'Oh, he couldn't cope with me complaining about my shoulder any more,' she said, almost impassively. Did I detect some sadness in her voice?

We spoke generally. Anne Marie just wanted to know how her years of toil in the swimming pool could have caused the shoulder problem, and how it in turn had caused the shake in her hand. She had not, she said, been on the internet, and this was clearly true, as she was not at all sure why she needed to see a neurologist.

'Well, should I have the shoulder surgery?' she asked.

I paused. It is shocking for a patient who thinks they have one fairly straightforward problem to be told that they have an altogether more serious one that they will have to live with for the rest of their lives. To diagnose in the first consultation without further tests is risky, lest it be something else and you lose the already unsettled patient's trust. But Anne Marie's surgery was scheduled for two weeks hence, so I didn't have the luxury of time to do tests or to introduce the concept of her condition gently. I was pretty sure, but not definite, that she had Parkinson's and it looked like I was going to have to tell her without the tests to confirm it.

In younger people like Anne Marie, we do blood tests and MRI scans and the more definitive dopamine transport (DAT) scan. This is a brain study in which the person is given iodine and a particular scan of their brain is performed. The area of the brain that would be affected by Parkinson's lights up when things are normal, but appears less bright on the scan if Parkinson's is present.

I said I wanted to arrange for tests, and that maybe she should postpone the surgery until I could be more sure.

'But why?' she asked. 'I've been in pain for ages and want to get on with my life. What difference will your tests make?'

Perfectly reasonable questions, and I could not avoid telling her.

'I think you may have an early form of Parkinson's disease,' I explained.

She blanched.

'That's an old person's disease. You must be wrong.' She started to sob.

I went through all the signs her body was displaying and did the foot-tapping trick. Her left leg was lacking the rhythm of the right, and when she saw it with her own eyes, she broke down. It was heartbreaking to see a relatively young woman observe her life fall apart.

You can only imagine where patients' thoughts go at a time like this. Unprepared patients can go into a trance-like state. Asking whether they have any questions is basically useless – most just want to run away from you to try and process what you have just told them. I will then get an email a day or two later, asking an array of questions. Typically it explains how they were too shocked at the time to take in anything I said. By this point they have been trawling the internet, further traumatizing themselves. The time of day the email is written is also telling, as are the typos – they are not thinking straight, and writing in the small hours of the morning when sleep is an impossibility.

Anne Marie, however, regained her composure quickly, which in itself was unusual. She dried her eyes, and said, 'OK, what's next?' I was taken aback at her apparent stoicism, but went through the tests I planned to arrange. I told her she should postpone the shoulder surgery. I promised to see her in a few weeks' time to clarify where we were once we had the results. She appeared to be listening, but I couldn't help but notice her mind seemed to have wandered.

I suggested that next time Anne Marie might bring her husband as support, and to help take in the information, but when she returned a few weeks later she was alone once again. The tests confirmed the diagnosis, and ruled out alternative possibilities. She definitely had Parkinson's.

It was discombobulating to see a completely different person in front of me when I went out to the waiting room to call Anne Marie into the office. She jumped up, smiled warmly and all but hugged me. I had spent a few sleepless hours the previous night myself worrying about how best to break the news. I had assumed there would be tears and perhaps some anger, but I got the opposite. She sat down and I said I wouldn't drag things out, and confirmed that the tests had shown that she did indeed have Parkinson's. We would have to start with medication and physiotherapy for her left arm and leg.

She smiled. 'Fair enough,' she said nonchalantly. 'Should we start dopamine now?'

'You seem to be taking this all very well,' I said. I asked, had something happened since I last saw her? 'I'm always keen to learn how someone turns bad news into good in their own head, both for myself and for patients in the future.'

'Well,' she said, still smiling, 'it's a funny thing, but this Parkinson's thing has been a bit of a blessing.'

Now that was a new one.

'I was devastated, initially, after our last meeting. But since then I've come to terms with it. I have been unhappy with my life for the last few years, and for the last six months I've been in contact with an old flame on Facebook. Myself and my husband had grown apart and I was constantly wondering if this was it. Everything felt stale. So, when the ex-boyfriend got in touch, it was exciting. There was a frisson. I won't lie: we had planned to meet up after the shoulder surgery. I was all set on having an affair with him.'

I was not following at all.

'So, how does all this make you seem almost . . . happy that you have Parkinson's?'

'I was planning on potentially wrecking my life . . . and my husband's . . . and my children's. I was going to risk everything for a stupid fling. I know that now. I looked around for the first time in years, and it was like I finally had my eyes opened. I began to realize how lucky I am. When I thought about all that I had to lose, I cancelled the rendezvous with my ex. I said nothing about the diagnosis. It doesn't matter to him.

'That's why I didn't bring my husband with me; I wanted to come to terms with the diagnosis on my own, to think about what life would be like with Parkinson's. I know he'll be there for me and I will bring him to the next appointment. So, basically, Parkinson's has kind of saved my life.'

It was one of the most uplifting and thought-provoking encounters I've ever had.

'Gunslinger's gait' was the term used by a group of researchers a few years ago to describe how ex-KGB men walked, with one arm swinging and one arm straight down by their side. Rumours on the internet suggested that President Vladimir Putin might be in the early stages of Parkinson's because, like Conor, the Russian president did not swing his right arm when he walked. Ultimately, the research team unearthed a KGB training manual that taught the agents to keep their right hand close to their chest while they were walking, the faster to draw their gun if threatened. When they looked back over the news footage for other possible signs of the condition, they soon debunked the myth that President Putin had Parkinson's.

The lesson was clear; regardless of the patient, it's an occupational hazard of neurologists that our training to hunt for clues can lead us to read too much into behaviours; without taking an adequate clinical history and, crucially, putting behaviour and history in context, a strong diagnosis isn't possible. I have diagnosed Parkinson's in someone sitting opposite me on a bus or a train, only to realize when they get up and walk off briskly that it's a Monday morning and their glum, expressionless face is merely showing how they feel about the week ahead.

Having said that, sometimes the signs of Parkinson's can be extraordinarily slight. I once met an engineer who, on retirement, was given a very fancy hi-tech watch. He wore it with pride and loved telling people how it was motion-sensitive; he joked that he knew he'd be dead if it ever stopped. Within a year of retirement, the watch stopped, but Mike was not dead. He brought it to be fixed, but they could find nothing wrong. It seemed to work well again for a while but then stopped again. Frustrated, he gave it to his son, thinking it might work better for someone else. His son wore the watch for two weeks, and sure enough, had no problems. He felt a twinge of conscience wearing his father's expensive gift, and returned it to his dad, telling him that he was imagining the faults. Mike wore it for a few more days, but once again it stopped.

Mike is the first and only person I have come across so far whose watch told me practically the exact time he had developed Parkinson's. The lack of movement in his left arm was indistinct but, like Conor, he was not moving the arm naturally when he walked, so his bradykinesia was such that the watch could not detect any motion. The onset of Parkinson's can be that subtle.

Of course, not every tremor turns out to be Parkinson's. Jason was eighteen when his mother, Yvonne, noticed that he had a problem. In fact, she heard it before she saw it. Jason was being the dutiful son, she thought wryly, bringing her a cup of tea while she watched *Downton Abbey* one Sunday evening. She was as specific as that because she was watching the screen rather than Jason and got distracted by the rattling of the cup on the saucer in his hand.

'What's wrong with you?' she said irritably. She assumed he was still recovering from his Saturday night excesses, having arrived home from 'gallivanting' at three in the morning. Jason assumed the same.

'Oh, stop giving me a hard time,' he said, and it blew over quickly.

Over the next few months, though, Jason began to notice that when he had indeed been out gallivanting, his hands were shaking a lot the next day. He googled 'shakes and hangover' and discovered the phrase delirium tremens (DTS).

'Oh God,' he thought, 'I'm an alcoholic.' He vowed to cut back on the booze, and he did.

The shaking improved for a while, but soon he realized that he'd shake under any pressure, particularly in front of the class at school. As time went on, the shaking was happening more and more, and now almost regardless of the social setting. It would go away when he was at rest, such as when he was watching television, but as soon as he tried to do anything that required a modicum of precision, like texting or writing, it would start again.

His second round of googling convinced him that he had Parkinson's, and he watched footage of Michael J. Fox on YouTube for a glimpse of what he thought would be his future self. He decided that he would die young, and that he might as well enjoy himself. So he went back to his late nights and boozy weekend binges. In fact, he quickly discovered that once he'd had three pints, his shaking hands were rocksteady once again – but the next morning the shakes were twice as bad as before.

It was at least six months before he told Yvonne. She looked at his outstretched hands trembling and recalled the cup and saucer rattling so loudly that night she was watching *Downton*. She recalled how her own mother had a shake in her hands most of her life, but it only caused her difficulties when she was in her seventies. She remembered being embarrassed when they were out and her mum would spill food down her front as she tried to bring a fork to her lips. Her mother had died ten years before from cancer, but she had wondered occasionally whether she had had undiagnosed Parkinson's.

Yvonne arranged to get Jason an appointment to see me. As it did not appear urgent from the GP's referral letter, the appointment was scheduled for some months hence. In the meantime, Jason's tremor was worsening. Yvonne was worried sick and shared her suspicions about their mother's shakes with her siblings.

'Oh, that's the family tremor,' her elder brother, Brian, told her. 'I have it, John has it, but Mary doesn't.' Relieved but confused, Yvonne wondered why no one had mentioned this 'family tremor' before, and how come she had never even noticed it in her brothers over all these years.

'Mine only started a few years ago, and only affects me from time to time so I just get on with it,' Brian said.

As a result of her detective work, Yvonne was calmed by the time she brought Jason in to see me. And it was indeed the case that he did not have Parkinson's. Instead, Jason had a type of shaking called a benign essential tremor. The benign bit and the tremor bit are self-explanatory, but the 'essential' part means, well, essentially nothing. We don't know what causes it exactly. (It is typical of us medics to come up with complicated explanations for questions we can't answer. We use 'idiopathic' and 'cryptogenic' a lot too, and again these terms mean, in essence, that we don't know what causes a condition or symptom.)

Such 'essential' tremors tend to run in families and are genetically referred to as autosomal-dominant, meaning that they are transmitted via our genes, so half of the patient's children might expect to be similarly affected. That said, essential tremors also have what is called variable penetrance, so can affect only one or two of a sufferer's children or may even skip a whole generation altogether.

The tremor is not, as in Parkinson's disease, present when the hands are at rest. It comes out when someone is performing a delicate task, like trying not to spill the tea; the cup rattling on the saucer can be a sign. It is made worse by stress, caffeine and, as with Jason, withdrawal from alcohol. 'So you're telling him he should give up booze altogether?' Yvonne asked, hopefully.

I explained that alcohol sometimes actually helps the shaking.

'So you're telling me I should drink more?' Jason jumped in.

It was funny to watch the mother–son interaction as they shot playful digs at each other through me. It was a relief to us all to share a laugh over such a relatively positive diagnosis.

Yet there was no cure for his shaking and the first thing we advise is to cut back on caffeine and alcohol – Yvonne clapped her hands in victory – 'particularly as many people in the past have become progressively more dependent on alcohol to overcome their shaking', I said.

Jason looked miserable, but cheered up when I reminded him that he did not have the Parkinson's he was worried about.

There are some drugs that we can use for this type of tremor. Often we use beta blockers, which work mainly by improving the body's receptors for rushes of adrenalin, the hormone that reacts to stimulating or anxious environments by making the heart go faster and putting you on edge. Beta blockers are familiar from their one-time prevalence in sport for helping with performance anxiety. Until they were largely prohibited, some sportspeople used these drugs in an attempt to control their shaking at critical moments; for instance, when they feared being unable to complete a shot in snooker, make a putt in golf or release a dart.

Generally, once someone is reassured that their shaking isn't part of the serious or fatal illness they feared, their anxiety subsides, and the tremor improves. And if they then avoid other provoking factors, things can improve even further. I tend to advise medication to help control a tremor only if it's substantially affecting their quality of life; the tablets I prescribe only mask the symptoms. Most of the people I have seen take the medication for a while, and then gradually wean themselves off it or take it only when there's cause for anxiety on the horizon – a father-of-the-bride speech is a common reason.

Martin's shaking came on when he was standing at a pedestrian crossing waiting for the green man. As the cars pulled up and Martin set off to cross the road towards his office he lost control of his body. He later described it as being like a bolt of lightning going through his body and, although it didn't hurt and he was fully conscious, he became frozen with the shock. Confused, he was roused from his very brief dream-like state by the car horns of the angry morning drivers. He realized he was standing in the middle of the road and the green man had turned red again.

'I must have blacked out,' he thought, but he was still standing and reasoned he would have fallen over if he had truly lost consciousness. He waved apologetically to the angry drivers and headed on into work.

He tried in vain to come up with anything he had done out of the ordinary, but despite his youth – he was just nineteen – Martin was a creature of habit and that weekend he hadn't ventured far from his usual set of bars and clubs. And though he had taken the occasional ecstasy tablet in the past, he hadn't taken anything that weekend.

He had a cup of coffee at work and looked at his colleagues in the hope that they wouldn't notice anything different about him. It seemed that they didn't, so Martin just went about his day. Still, he was deeply disturbed by this 'bolt of lightning' and for the next few days worried he was coming down with something. It was with some trepidation that he came up to the same traffic lights on the mornings that followed. When nothing further happened, he decided he must have imagined the whole thing.

Weeks later he set out on his evening run. Martin was a fit young man who had already finished three Dublin marathons and planned to do Boston the following spring. He did a few stretches and closed the door of his flat behind him. Just a few steps from the door he lost control of his body again. He appeared to be having, he thought, some sort of fit. He stood stock-still, and the twitching movements subsided, but when he took some tentative steps, it happened again. He was sure he faced an early death.

He was grateful that no one had seen this fit, which was as brief as the first. He went back into his apartment, took off his runners and fired up his computer. He googled 'fits' and 'epilepsy' and decided this was the problem. He recalled a distant cousin who had epilepsy, but his cousin's seizures were like the ones he saw on television medical dramas, and Martin's weren't like that.

His head was full of questions: *'What will I tell my folks?'*, *'Will I lose my job?'*, *'Will I be able to drive?'* – the websites all pointed out that epilepsy could severely restrict your chances of getting a driving licence – *'Am I going insane?'*

He ran through the gamut of possible neurological diseases as he scrolled. 'Oh God, I have Parkinson's. Or multiple sclerosis.' Finally, 'I have motor neuron disease' – the searches nearly always end with motor neuron disease. But Martin kept going until he came across a blog about Huntington's disease. The blogger's description of his involuntary movements seemed to match his own experience, though Martin's twitches were brief and passing.

He closed his laptop and started to cry. His life was over. He would never run the Boston marathon. Suddenly his hopes and expectations of life narrowed down to crossing his fingers and praying to God that he wouldn't end up in a wheelchair.

When Martin came in to see me the dark circles around his eyes testified to his sleepless nights. He came to see me alone and, perhaps having watched too many fast-talking TV medical shows, he explained his problem at speed. After a few short minutes, he caught his breath, looked at me grimly and said, 'Give it to me straight, Doc. Don't sugar-coat it. I can handle it.'

I felt so sorry for him but I struggled to stifle a smile at his Americanisms, gleaned from a combination of *Grey's Anatomy* and *House*, and his attempt to simulate what so-called 'brave patients' are supposed to sound like. There was no family history of Huntington's, and the only person with a neurological problem he knew of was his second cousin with epilepsy. He didn't smoke, and was very healthy apart from his weekend binge-drinking and the occasional ecstasy tablet. I examined him and could find nothing untoward, so reassured him that I did not think he had MS, Parkinson's or MND.

After a heartfelt sigh of relief and shedding a brief tear, he said, 'So, am I going mad?'

It had crossed my mind, and I do see a lot of deeply anxious young people, but I kept that to myself. I explained that I would request some tests and I asked him to keep a record of further attacks while we looked into it.

'But what if it happens again? Is there no medication you can give me?'

As I didn't know what I was treating, I couldn't yet offer a solution. Crestfallen, despite having been reassured that his worst fears were unfounded, he left the clinic room angry and deeply unhappy. He was sure I didn't believe him, and I didn't know how to convince him that I did.

I expedited all his tests, and within a few weeks he was back in my office.

'It's happened at least ten times since I saw you last. I kept the diary you asked me to, and the only time it definitely doesn't happen is when I'm watching TV or am in bed.'

He showed me the diary and his extensive notes. 'Monday afternoon, bolt of lightning when out walking to lunch with colleagues . . . Thursday morning, halfway across the road on way to work . . . Saturday morning, two minutes into my run . . .' And on it went. 'It seems when I'm still, I'm fine, but when I move, my body can sometimes go into a spasm like I'm possessed, but not every time.'

His scans and electrical test were all clear. He exhaled, not with relief but with frustration. 'So, I am going mad then,' he said.

I had seen just a handful of these cases over twenty-five years in neurology, and mainly such patients were presented at 'grand rounds', when rare conditions are presented to a group of neurologists, especially if the treating physician is unsure of what is wrong or what to do next. It is a cornerstone of neurology, and is both highly stimulating for the doctors and in most cases also extremely helpful for the patients.

Martin had a condition called paroxysmal kinesigenic choreathetosis (PKC). It was first documented in the early twentieth century in London in two patients with intermittent involuntary movements, like those Martin described, and the unusual spasmodic flailing is brought on by the initiation of voluntary movement. There have been many reports of similar cases since, and this odd excessive movement disorder (*hyper*kinetic as opposed to *hypo*kinetic or reduced movements, as with Parkinson's) generally begins in childhood. There have been reports of it running in families (though, to his knowledge, it didn't in Martin's). We don't know why or how involuntary movements happen, but it has been suggested it may be a problem with the channels lining the nerves of affected people. More simply, it's thought that the wires moving our arms and legs have faults – often inherited – that affect transmission of signals from the brain.

It must be very strange to non-medics at times when we describe conditions like this that we know so little about. Inevitably, 'dodgy wiring' doesn't cut it as an explanation for someone as curious as Martin, who fears his life is threatened, but sometimes that is the best and only thing we can come up with. People expect doctors to make a diagnosis and then be able to explain the mechanics involved before starting to treat them. Yet medicine is still something of an art; with a condition like Martin's, it's a question of listening, observing and tracking the patterns of disease, then formulating a diagnosis from the pieces of the puzzle.

I was excited about Martin's diagnosis; I explained that his life was not at risk, and that there was a treatment for the disorder. We use anti-epileptic drugs for a range of conditions: neuralgia, certain pain syndromes and even some movement disorders associated with MS. I prescribed one of these drugs at a very low dose for Martin and asked him to keep his diary as before. In spite of his understandable scepticism, given the slim information and the lack of other options, he tried the tablets. Within four weeks, the movements had stopped and he was back training for the Boston marathon.

I followed him up for a few years, but he got tired of coming to see me once the movements had gone away, and his GP could renew his prescription. I see him from time to time around the city socializing with friends but we haven't spoken. It may be that he doesn't recognize me, or doesn't want to recognize me; either way it appears that what he thought of as his brush with mortality is a distant memory. That's all you really can strive for when trying to repatriate people to the land of the well.

32

DOCTORING IN THE TWENTY-FIRST CENTURY

Doctors once seemed to have so much time to chat. Now it seems every moment of every working day has to be accounted for and patients (and, indeed, doctors) are more like numbers on a spreadsheet than people with complex stories that are the backdrop to their ailments. Knowing where a person is from, not just geographically but psychologically and emotionally, can frame how they might perceive their symptoms and their reactions to them. Taking the time to listen – to, say, how a relative who had a distressing time in hospital has instilled a subconscious fear of doctors – can reveal a lot more than a patient's physical complaints.

Time is the enemy of such interactions these days. We have a thing called KPIS – key performance indicators – where we are asked, for example, to see a set minimum number of patients each day; to try to discharge people as early as is safe from hospital to free up the bed for the next person waiting on a trolley; or to reduce the waiting-list times by seeing more people in less time. These are all eminently understandable goals, but I fear that they can miss the point of what we are trying to do. Previously the only 'KPI' was whether you were doing your best to get the patients under your care well and return them home. We still do that, of course, but try to do so for twice as many people in half the time. It can be emotionally exhausting for doctors and, I imagine, it must seem much less caring to the patients.

I suspect trying to maintain the precarious balance between efficiency and empathy is one of the main reasons for doctors burning out. Everybody has a finite reserve of empathy and no one can possibly get on with everyone they meet. Working under pressure it is easy to see how difficult communications – and many communications in a medical setting are difficult – aren't handled as sensitively as they might be. And a wrong word can cause antipathy bordering on resentment.

It is a great privilege to look after people. Traditionally medicine has been perceived as being a high-prestige profession and doctors have benefited from that. But it is not always an easy job. It is interesting to note how aware we are becoming – finally, and at a snail's pace – of the need for doctors to look after themselves. It is draining to try to stay in intellectual control while your day is an emotional rollercoaster. As a neurologist you can meet, back to back, patients in dramatically different circumstances – one whose problem you can resolve easily and another to whom you are giving a death sentence. You must stay inquisitive, analytical and, crucially, as kind as you can be when faced with either individual.

Reading a patient's emotions takes years of practice, meaning that doctors get it wrong for years, too. On top of that, a doctor will only have about thirty minutes (or less) to assess a patient's entire life, how it has been changed by the illness and how that illness will affect those around them. Then the doctor not only has to come up with a diagnosis, which may affect the patient for ever, but has also to try to reassure and comfort them.

Every word must be chosen carefully, as it will be picked over again later. Like all doctors, and regardless of my best intentions, I get it wrong at times: I will be too serious and arrogant for some, and too light-hearted and flippant for others. Choosing the wrong word can take away the patient's sense of hope, or make them feel that you are attempting to control their life. Though apologizing for a misstep is awkward, failing to pick up on a patient being upset is worse. You can hear about it through the grapevine and it's dispiriting, both personally and professionally.

During the banking crisis in Ireland a few years ago, I saw many patients who worked in the banks at various levels. They would admit to their occupation rather diffidently as the banks were then public enemy number one. I saw quite a few young bank workers at that time. They presented with a wide variety of complaints, mostly headaches. Regardless of their status in the bank, they told me awful stories of how customers would treat them. Tellers said that they would be routinely abused by customers of all ages and from all walks of life. Even the security guards would get nasty comments as they opened the bank's doors each morning.

At the time, there was a deep sense of anger and betrayal in the country, and understandably so, given the widespread suffering caused by the banks' misdeeds and the resulting financial crisis. People listened to tales of management ineptitude and, sometimes, outright deceit, on the news, and were enraged. And it seems many considered any bank employee fair game. As a result of this misdirected fury, the bank's staff were getting sick. These stressed young men and women came to me with severe migraines, tremors, pins and needles and chronic insomnia, among other complaints. I cannot recall diagnosing any of them with anything serious, but all were under extreme pressure.

I think about this state of affairs when I hear yet another news item about the health service. In a similar way to the bank workers, hospital staff can be treated appallingly. I don't suggest that things are ideal in the health service – far from it. Nor would I try to pretend that mistakes don't happen. It is totally appropriate that patients demand much of their doctors and nurses; after all, they are dealing with matters of life and death. But the sense among people when shortcomings become manifest that we are all in it together – doctors, nurses, patients, and all of our families and friends – no longer seems to prevail. With rising trolley counts, and delays getting people out of hospital because of insufficient resources in the community, a 'them and us' mentality seems to have taken hold and set some vocal patients against hospital staff. It is thankfully only a minority of people who take this approach, but those who shout loudest tend to get the most attention as we defensively try to appease them, neglecting the quiet ones in need around them.

Aggressive patients, though a tiny minority, have a terrible effect on doctors and nurses who are doing their utmost to be courteous while giving their best care. Of course, some people are so scared by their diagnosis or the treatments involved that they lash out, but this doesn't account for all of it. And it's not just doctors and nurses who are at the receiving end of mistreatment, but medical secretaries and other support staff too. I've seen colleagues in every area being reduced to tears by the abuse meted out by some patients.

As in most walks of life, it is the 5 per cent of people who take up 95 per cent of our time who we think – and fret – about most. Instead of celebrating the good work we do and the patients who are satisfied by our care, we spend an inordinate amount of time worrying about the 5 per cent. This small but vociferous minority of dissatisfied patients frequently warns us that our perceived shortcomings will be exposed in the media, particularly on Joe Duffy's *Liveline* – 'I'll talk to Joe' is a common threat; 'I'll destroy your reputation' is another. Such threats serve to make doctors over-investigative as a defence against potential accusations of malpractice. This helps no one, particularly not an already over-burdened public health system.

In more extreme scenarios, things can take a nasty turn. I once called the gardaí because a series of abusive emails, culminating in threats to myself and my family, began to seriously disturb me. This was after two years of doing everything I could to help a young man who would not believe that I was not out to do anything but harm to him. He was mentally unstable, but I had no recourse other than going to the gardaí; taking him to court would have been heavy-handed and embarrassingly public for us both. The gardaí had a word with him and he backed off.

Doctors and nurses don't expect unquestioning trust. We listen to the evening news and follow the newspaper reports of health service mismanagement and medical disasters as closely as everyone else, if not more. We too have our own fears, rages and frustrations at the imperfections of the system in which we work. But a lack of basic respect from a minority of our patients can make many in the health service feel even more demoralized.

It is such a privilege to hear someone's life story and discuss openly how various social factors might be affecting their physical health. It is great when we can smile, chat, share a laugh with patients, even in grim situations, and comfort them when they are fearful. It serves to remind both sides of our common humanity – which is ultimately what we all need to hold on to as we get through the most difficult times, together.

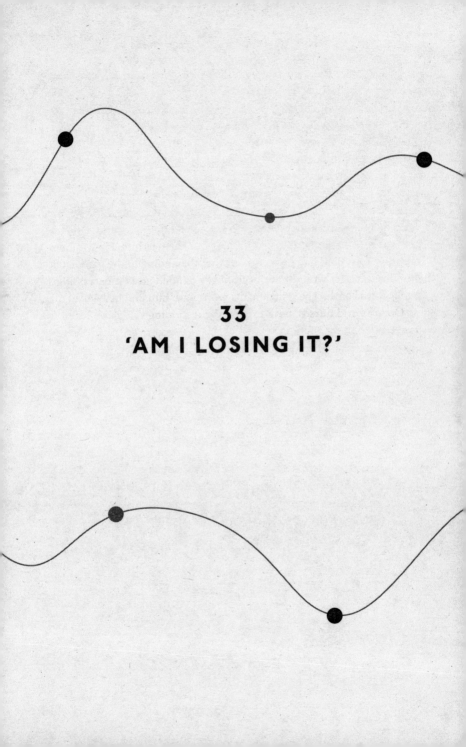

33
'AM I LOSING IT?'

I recently awoke at around three in the morning, and could not remember the lead guitarist of the Rolling Stones, a band I have loved for years. Nothing. Not even that behemoth of excess . . . what was his name? Had this rock star been replaced in the musical jukebox of my memory by someone else? Beyoncé? Rihanna? Surely not? Might Keith Richards' name assume less importance with time, dropping down the charts in my hippocampus? Or do we each have finite space for such memories? When I thought about it I wondered how medical students – who have to learn not just about neurology, but cardiology, the respiratory system, gastroenterology and a whole curriculum on surgery – ever cope? How had I coped?

In worrying about our memory we're all in the same boat, regardless of circumstances. The addled parent keeping an eye on the children while trying to prepare dinner and wondering how they're going to get a presentation finished in time for work the next day will inevitably drop the memory ball now and again. Everyone has experienced losing their keys once in a while, or being unable to find their car in a supermarket car park. We jokingly refer to them as 'senior moments'. Yet, if there is a family history of neurological conditions, perfectly healthy people worry that their quite ordinary human lapses in memory are the tip of the iceberg of dementia. Anxiety grows, silently at first, exacerbating their inability to concentrate, causing more memory problems and fuelling their panic about a neurodegenerative disease. Our minds are all so cluttered in this age of information, and we are so constantly and actively interrupted by competing demands on our time, that it is hard to delineate where routine forgetfulness ends and true cognitive impairment begins.

I see at least four or five people a week who are worried about their failing memory. They will usually have experience of a parent or grandparent with dementia. And I will know within a few minutes that I'll be able to send them home happy; if they have kept their appointment, travelled to see me alone, given a precise story about their concerns and – ironically – faithfully recalled their memory lapses, the chances are they are perfectly healthy.

Yet even once I have performed the basic cognitive assessments

('Who is the president? Where are we? What day is it?'), it can be very difficult to persuade them that there's no great likelihood of there being any cause for concern. So we proceed. 'Please draw the face of a clock, and put the hands to tell the time at ten past eleven. Give me as many words beginning with the letter F as you can in a minute,' and I smile, 'but no names or expletives, please.' It's eye-opening to see a worried person react to these simple tasks under the pressure of a doctor's gaze. They will focus exclusively on their one or two mistakes, regardless of my reassurance; a truly unwell patient puts all of the clock face numbers down one side of the page, or lists only a few F words in the allocated minute. The latter rarely needs me to point out that there's something seriously wrong.

There is still no definitive test for Alzheimer's. Instead, as is frequently the case in neurology, we try to piece together the jigsaw of the problem. At times, even the diagnostic tools we have leave doctors still sitting on the fence when we see someone making heavy weather of these basic tasks. A fear of labelling someone wrongly – a misdiagnosis – is obviously a major concern for medical reasons, but on a more human level telling someone they have Alzheimer's is shattering, and may lead to depression and social withdrawal, which can further accentuate any cognitive problems. Would you want to know you had a condition for which the medical treatment is, at best, limited? If you did, what would you do about it? If we live long enough, a substantial proportion of us will eventually develop at least a degree of cognitive decline, yet we still discuss dementia in hushed tones, as if by not talking about it, it might go away. It won't.

Emma was an old friend from London who had moved back to Dublin with her husband and two children. Her mother had died of breast cancer when Emma was only fifteen and her brother about eighteen. Emma and I were close and had spent many a wild night out in Soho when I lived there. She felt terrible about pursuing her career as an architect in London while her father lived alone, and had promised him she would return to Dublin as soon as it was feasible.

We lost touch for a few years while I was working in Paris and Melbourne, but when I returned to Ireland, I was glad to hear that Emma had been back for a few years herself, and we arranged to meet. My first thought when Emma arrived at the café was that she looked exhausted. I forgot about that as we got to catching up and she told me how she had fallen in love, got married and then become pregnant soon after I had left London. Her husband was a fellow Dubliner and they quickly made the decision to move home.

'My dad was delighted, of course,' Emma told me. 'I had gone home at least twice a year over the years to see him, and we still got on really well, so I was looking forward to spending more time with him.'

Emma's father, Peter, was now in his mid-sixties and was about to retire from his job lecturing in architecture.

'He loved his buildings, and it was like a guided tour of Dublin when we went for our walks together when I was back, but he had no other hobbies,' Emma said. 'He played poker with a few old cronies on Tuesday nights and maybe had dinner with some sympathetic couples once a week, but otherwise he was alone in the world. I knew he'd be thrilled to have the grandkids and myself back, but I was worried he would become too dependent on us.

'It was fine when we were back initially. If I'm honest, it gave us a chance to reintegrate socially as we had a babysitter on tap. Simon and myself could go out a lot more often than we might have without him around, so that was brilliant.

'When Dad did retire, it was like a switch went off. He seemed lost and didn't know what to do with himself. He would call around in the morning and offer to take the kids to school. He was spending more time with the kids than we were. He would come around for tea and turn up unannounced for Sunday lunch. I tried to set him up with some widowed mothers of friends, but he always said he would never meet anyone like Mum, and nothing came of his dates.

'It was a lot of exposure after years of being independent in London and we had a row one Christmas. I shouted at him to back off a bit. He was heartbroken but, Dad being Dad, was very understanding. He more or less withdrew from our lives for a few months. In no time, the sense of guilt got the better of me and I called around to his place. He was in a desperate state and the house was pure chaos. There was food everywhere and he even looked like he had stopped washing himself.

'He was lonely and depressed, and it was my fault. I felt terrible and I tried to undo the damage and invited him around again all the time, but it wasn't the same. He seemed to have lost interest in life. He would babysit occasionally, but the joy was gone out of it for him. He seemed so unhappy, and started to snap at the kids, whom he adored.

'When he forgot to pick up Charlie from school one day, I began to realize something might be wrong, but I didn't know how to approach it. I persuaded him to see his GP, who agreed he was depressed and suggested a referral to a psychiatrist. Dad refused to go; he didn't trust doctors after Mum had died so young – sorry.' She smiled when I flinched.

'So we muddled along for a year like that, but I lost confidence in his ability to mind the kids and he noticed that I was asking him over to mind them less and less. He agreed to let me hire a cleaner, which helped for a while. I thought he was coming out of his post-retirement blues but then I met one of his poker buddies in Tesco.

'Jim asked me how Dad was. "What do you mean?" I said, "Sure, you see him every Tuesday?" He told me he hadn't been coming since January. It was June then, and Dad hadn't said a thing about not going to poker any more. Jim seemed wary so I asked if they'd had an argument or something.

'He said it was nothing like that, just that Dad didn't seem to enjoy the cards as much and didn't seem to be able to concentrate on the game at times. "We were worried he was drinking a bit too much," he said, "but we didn't like to say anything. And then he just stopped coming." Jim said he called him a few times to ask him over but Dad said he was babysitting. So, after a while, he just stopped asking.

'I was shocked but kept it together in front of Jim and decided to confront Dad at the weekend. When I called to the house it was in a state again. I called the cleaner to vent but she told me Dad had informed her months before that he didn't need her any longer.

'When I asked Dad about it, he said he didn't want anyone in his house and he could look after himself. "But, Dad," I said, "you can't. Look around you."

'He started to cry, and it was the first time since Mum died that I had seen him cry. You have no idea how upsetting it is to see your father cry.'

At this point in the story, Emma was crying herself. Over the following few months, she renewed her efforts to include her father in her family's coming and goings. She brought him with them on family trips to the zoo, the Botanic Gardens and even took him shopping, which she knew he hated but felt it would at least get him out of the house. Nothing was helping. Peter was uninterested in everything, and when he came around to their house would sit quietly in the corner nursing a glass of whiskey.

She thought the problem might be booze, but she didn't think he drank that much. Nonetheless, she asked him to cut back, causing another almighty argument. 'How dare you?' he had shouted at her. 'Mind your own business, just like you've done most of your life since your mum died. Why are you trying to make amends now?'

Emma was destroyed by blaming herself. She called her brother in Sydney, even though he was too far away to help. He and their father had fallen out years earlier over something no one could now remember, but his anger hadn't abated, so her efforts fell flat.

Emma went with her father to their family doctor once more, and when the GP recommended that he see a neurologist, she knew there must be something more to all of this.

It is remarkable how even close families can miss what is right in front of their eyes. When I met Peter it was nearly two years since his retirement. Emma had told me he was always rather reserved but the man before me was barely able to look me in the eye. He sat down and then, just as quickly, stood up to take off his coat. He became flustered looking for a coat hook, and then irritated when I asked him how old he was. Emma was mortified.

'Just tell him how old you are,' she said.

'Nineteen forty-two,' he said sullenly.

'How old does that make you?' I asked.

'You're the doctor. If you're so smart, you can work it out.'

'Dad!' Emma said. 'What's wrong with you? Don't be so rude.'

'There's nothing wrong with me!' he said, loudly. 'You're the one dragging me along to see this quack.'

There was an awkward pause as Emma looked at me in shock, red-faced. This was the moment she understood that her father was no longer the man he used to be. He had always been kind and gentle, her hero all her life. But his changed character could no longer be denied. She didn't need a neurologist to tell her something was seriously wrong with her father's brain.

Reluctantly, Peter finally answered a few of my basic questions, but baulked at my request to draw a clock. 'Don't treat me like a child,' he fumed.

I asked him about his favourite buildings in Dublin, and which ones he might recommend I see; I admitted I knew nothing about architecture. He softened a little, but stalled.

'The main ones,' he said.

'Can you give me an example?' I asked.

'You know the ones I mean,' he replied tersely.

I moved on to the physical examination. He shuffled when he walked, but it wasn't Parkinson's. His feet appeared stuck to the floor; it's called 'marche à petit pas' (walking with small steps) and suggests the involvement of the frontal lobes of the brain. Problems in this area can also affect our emotional state.

When I placed my fingers in his hands he grasped them reflexively, like a child does when you place your finger in their tiny palms. I scratched the belly of his thumb muscle gently and the side of his mouth (mentalis muscle) contracted. When I placed the knuckle of my index finger on his lips he pursed as if to kiss it. Peter was showing many of the neurological signs we see in children before their frontal lobes develop. When the front part of the brain develops, the so-called primitive reflexes I was eliciting disappear. When it starts to degenerate or atrophy, these primitive reflexes may reappear. In other words, a part of Peter's brain had gone back to its 'baby state'. He had frontal lobe dementia. Emma started to cry quietly. Peter put his arm around her, and his eyes welled up too.

While there are different types of dementia, by far the most common is Alzheimer's disease. Regardless of type, it involves the slow degeneration of one's cognitive faculties, usually starting with memory, and is often associated with behavioural changes. In the initial stages it is extremely variable between individual patients; some become docile and withdrawn while others appear agitated or even belligerent.

Our ability to treat dementia is still very limited. Medications can – sometimes – slow the cognitive decline somewhat, but it would be a brave doctor who would give a definitive answer to the inevitable question of 'How long?' The truth is that we just do not know with any certainty exactly how each person will decline, but decline they will. Some seem fine or at least functional for years; others only get months.

I arranged scans and blood tests just in case there was a more treatable cause of Peter's memory problems, to check vitamin levels and thyroid function and to exclude tumours that can fool us, but I knew I was just trying to put off the inevitable conversation with my old friend. The MRI scan showed that Peter's brain had begun to atrophy (shrink) already, and Emma called a halt to further tests; she knew they wouldn't change anything.

Practical to a fault, Emma arranged an enduring power of attorney order and started to research nursing homes. It was still early days, but Peter was already coming to the point where he could not safely live alone any longer. Until she found somewhere, Emma wondered if she could manage him in her own home with her husband and young children. She didn't want him to go into a nursing home: 'They're all so depressing,' she told me. 'I feel like I'm just getting rid of him after all he has done for me,' she said. 'Is it awful for me to wish he would die peacefully in the night?'

Peter refused to move into Emma's, so for a year or more she juggled her job, her marriage and her children with what she referred to as 'her latest child' – her father. Something had to give, and eventually she took some time off work. When I met her on one of her now very rare nights off, she was a shadow of her former self. Her upset at Peter's diagnosis had been replaced by feeling guilty for having persuaded him to go into a nursing home, which he had eventually done. Now she was angry. 'Why me?' she lamented. There was nothing useful that I, or anyone, could say. All of us feel useless to some extent in the face of dementia, and as a doctor it is depressing not to be able to help much either.

'It's like bringing up another child – in reverse,' she told me. 'He can't dress himself. He makes a huge mess every time he tries to eat, and we more or less have to feed him. His steps are as tentative as when the children were learning to walk. When we have him out for a visit and he goes to get up, just to go into the kitchen, we all hold our breath and, if he even sways slightly, someone will jump up to prevent him falling. It's like he's been trapped in his adult brain his whole life, and now he's as dependent as he was as a small child, and he can't remember any of it. He behaves like a child too, either sulky or happy.

'How did the same brain grow from nothing as a child, to develop over a lifetime, only to disintegrate back to what he started with near the end? At least with cancer or heart disease you could blame his lifestyle but here there's nothing. There's no reason to it. He has always been very healthy, and he used to lecture me about drinking and smoking when I was younger. What's the point?'

Emma was already mourning her father, and mourning the living brings with it many of the same mixed emotions as mourning the dead. She was sad for him, but she also felt sorry for herself – and scared for the future. Will this happen to me? Will it happen to my children? We try to show empathy, to grieve for our loved ones when they get sick or die, but a lot of our grief is for ourselves and our own fate.

Peter lived in the nursing home for another four years. For the first couple of years Emma would bring him out for a walk, or even attempt a lunch in a local restaurant. But eventually she gave up on this. Her children were growing up. She returned to work, and life took over again. Her father acknowledged her less and less when she called in to see him. By the end, he didn't recognize Emma or his grandchildren. People talk about flickers of recognition in their loved ones suffering from dementia, but Emma saw none of this. Her visits tailed off.

By the time her father died, Emma was emotionally spent. 'He died three years before he died,' she told me later. She would suffer waves of guilt for a very long time after he had passed away. It was only years later that she was able to think of him again as the father he had been, the kind man who had done his best for her after her mother died, putting aside his own broken heart. She remembered his loving soliloquies about his work and how much that had inspired her. Finally, instead of being haunted by the vacant shell he had become, she was able to miss her lovely father, and mourn both him and the lost years at the end of his life.

34
'WHERE DO ALL THE OLD PEOPLE GO?'

'Where do all the old people go?' my young nephew once asked me, wide-eyed with disbelief when he discovered that his uncle looked after sick people.

'What do you mean?'

'Well, I know that people get sick and some of them die – but not all of them? So where do the ones who don't die go?'

I wasn't sure what to say. And for all of the childish naïveté of the question it struck me that his understanding wasn't all that far removed from how many of us proceed through life, somehow not quite grasping that death is coming for us all. Indeed, I sometimes wonder: what do people think is going to happen to them, ultimately?

The older I get as a doctor – and, indeed, as a potential patient of the future – the more that thoughts of a 'good death' occupy me. Is there such a thing? We hear of men and women who have sudden heart attacks and die in their beds and, while the shock is hard to overcome, it is frequently, according to their surviving loved ones, a great relief that they did not suffer.

Yet the expectation of their being a cure for everything and everyone is a strange defence mechanism we employ to avoid thinking about the inevitability of our own death. When people bring their elderly relatives to hospital, how much do they want the doctors to put their loved ones through before saying enough is enough? Obviously, we treat everyone as best we can and aim to restore the optimum quality of life for everyone regardless of age – after all, some eighty-year-olds look and act like fifty-year-olds, and vice versa, so age in years is not necessarily an indication of well-being or even health. You always want to give people hope. But when do you stop giving false hope and face reality?

Patients' families can be annoyed when a doctor suggests that someone may only have weeks to live, as if they are 'giving up' on them. Likewise, they feel vindicated when a patient defies all predictions and lives to see another year or more. The flip side, of course, is worse – when you suggest someone should be fine and then within days they die of a complication of their illness that was impossible to predict.

Modern medicine is exalted by most free-thinking folk. The progress in research and treatments in the last fifty years has been exhilarating, and the strides made to keep us alive at either end of life are astounding. Have we, however, reached the zenith of life preservation at one end of the scale? Are we keeping people alive for our sakes, or for theirs?

As doctors, many of us say we would like to be treated differently from the way we treat our own patients, which strikes me as curious. We likely say it because we see many relatives who are oddly willing to inflict painful tests and the misery of waiting on results on people who are coming to their natural end. Or when we propose that a course of treatment be stopped, there will always be one family member who will disagree, putting you and the other family members in the invidious position of having to keep someone alive and possibly in distress against your better nature. Most doctors have seen the traumatic deaths of frail, elderly and infirm patients and never want to go through something similar themselves.

This is what happens. If a person in the terminal stages of life does not have a Do Not Resuscitate (DNR) order clearly outlined in their medical notes, then it is incumbent on the nursing staff to call the emergency cardiac arrest team when someone suddenly deteriorates. This involves a team of doctors from all around the hospital getting paged simultaneously, dropping whatever they are doing and rushing to the patient who has possibly arrested.

It is rather frightening to see a horde of young doctors running along corridors past people sitting having coffee with visitors, a stark reminder to those who are less sick of what can be at stake in hospital. It is even more upsetting for the elderly men or women in a geriatric ward to see a group of frantic young doctors trying to bring someone they may know back from the dead. We try to protect the other patients from seeing such things but it is not always possible as the team tries to attach drips, set up the cardiac monitoring machine and begin the electrical attempts to restart a stopped heart.

Sometimes the effort is successful; other times the arrest team is not able to resuscitate the poor patient and, after an hour or more of chaos on the ward, the old men or women must try and go back to sleep as their erstwhile roommate is taken to the morgue. It is the stuff of nightmares. It is because we have all seen this so many times that doctors say we do not want this to happen to ourselves or our loved ones. Of course, maybe we will change our minds when it is our turn.

We often offer families of the infirm elderly the option of a DNR order if the chances of a meaningful recovery seem extremely limited. By meaningful we mean that we hope to resuscitate everyone, but not at the expense of brain damage or physical incapacity that might leave them in a worse state than before the arrest team was called. If someone's heart stops beating for long enough, then the brain becomes severely damaged and, while we might restore a heartbeat, we might not restore their mental faculties.

Some patients are resigned in the face of illness and will tell you frankly what they do and do not want in terms of treatment. Others will go into a deep state of denial or anger when the treatment appears not to be working. At such times it is hard not to countenance your own mortality, and that of your own loved ones.

Ultimately, 'Where do all the old people go?' has only one answer, and I think people are becoming more aware that they should be having this conversation earlier in their lives, rather than burying their heads in the sand.

Abigail was ninety-three years old when I was called to see her. She had been in hospital for nearly three months with pneumonia and had started shaking when she was eating her dinner. It had taken the reduced staff that long to notice because for the first two months Abigail was unable to feed herself.

She had been diagnosed with dementia a year or two before, and had refused to go into a nursing home when her friends had suggested it. She lived in a second-floor apartment with a lift, so somehow she had managed to look after herself prior to her admission to hospital. She had a son, Geoffrey, who lived in Norway with his family and was not home in Ireland much.

When I approached Abigail's bedside I saw the frailest woman I had ever seen up to that point. She looked like a little bird, her hair an unruly mass of long grey tresses. She lay so still on her bed while the ward bustled around her I presumed she was asleep. It was like seeing a once-famous movie star in repose. I coughed and she opened one eye to look at me suspiciously.

'Hello,' I said quietly and introduced myself. I addressed her by her formal name and she said, 'I'm Abigail, and I don't go in for any of that title nonsense.'

'OK, Abigail,' I said, 'I'm one of the doctors here and I have been asked to see you about the shake you have in your hand. Do you mind chatting to me for a while? Perhaps I can help.'

She looked at me quizzically, as if trying to get the measure of me. She seemed suspicious but patted the bed beside her indicating where I should sit.

From her medical notes I knew that in the lead-up to her admission she had not answered her phone for a day or two, so one of her friends had called around. When there was no answer to the doorbell a neighbour had let her into Abigail's flat. The place was in chaos. Newspapers dating back years were strewn around as well as boxes of photographs and letters from her younger days. The bins were overflowing and there was food rotting in the small fridge that caused an unpleasant odour throughout the apartment.

Abigail was in bed and had no idea who her friend was, so an ambulance was called to bring her to Casualty. The doctors confirmed she had severe pneumonia, and she was admitted to the geriatric ward, in a six-bedded bay with other elderly women around her. Her friends were told the outlook was not good and her son had been called to ask him to come home from Norway.

Geoffrey arrived two days later. The doctors told him that they did not think she was strong enough to survive the infection. They would do everything they could, but advised that he prepare himself for the worst.

He was furious. 'What do you mean?' he shouted. 'She just has a chest infection. Surely you can treat that. They certainly could do better in Norway.'

(Geoffrey's reaction is not uncommon. With our mighty diaspora, we often find it is the people who are farthest away from Ireland who want to have the most input when their parents become ill. It's something of an Irish solution to an Irish problem, as grown children, feeling the effects of guilt, homesickness and helplessness, weigh in on the family crisis. This may take the form of a critique of the Irish health service. If they live in any kind of developed country, as far as they are concerned the care where they are living is always better than that in Ireland.)

The doctors pointed out to Geoffrey that they had spoken to his mother's friends, who had outlined Abigail's steady decline over the preceding year or two. She was confused at times about where she was, and even who they were.

'Nonsense,' he said. 'I've spoken to her on the phone and she sounded fine to me. She must have been developing the pneumonia when they saw her like that. I want everything that can be done to be done.'

After a few days of similar conversations the doctors could not persuade Geoffrey that perhaps the end was near for his mother and acquiesced to his wishes.

They had already started antibiotics but the doctors had asked Geoffrey – her legal next of kin – whether they should have a DNR order in Abigail's notes in the event that she were to deteriorate rapidly. Geoffrey was adamant about not allowing one to be put in place.

As it was, Abigail was not in a position to give her own opinion. She thought she was still at home when I sat down beside her. We discussed her life and she could recall some of her earlier years. She told me about the grand dances she used to attend in London years before. She could not tell me what day it was ('What does it matter?') or even what year ('Oh, they all blur into one at my stage in life . . .') and I quickly understood I was irritating her with my incessant questions.

She brightened up when the tea arrived, but expressed dismay at the lack of saucers and the absence of a proper teapot. I saw her little hand shake as she lifted the mug to her lips. She had developed some of the early symptoms of Parkinson's in addition to her dementia. Medication would help but I did not tell her what I was thinking. Giving someone like Abigail a label with a name she might recognize, like Parkinson's, can be more morale-sapping than helpful.

I listened to Abigail's stories for a while but gradually she slipped back into her own world and soon fell asleep. The pneumonia was almost cleared, her doctors told me. She should be able to go home soon. But home to what?

I met some of her friends when they visited and was struck by their loyalty and sense of responsibility towards their cherished friend. For a woman of such senior years she was surrounded by a surprising number of friends, many of whom were many years younger than her. Before her decline in the year or so before she was hospitalized, they got in the habit of calling in to keep her company. They would bring her food on the pretext that they had cooked too much for their own families. Occasionally they would bring her out to a fancy restaurant, and Abigail would always insist on paying her own way. She was a woman of significant means whose husband had died when they were in their fifties, so Abigail had been living on her own for nearly forty years and was fiercely independent.

One woman showed me photographs of Abigail as a younger woman. Those old grey tresses had once been blonde and Abigail was strikingly beautiful. She had lived a glamorous life and had travelled extensively both before and after her husband's death. She knew many famous people, and her friends told me of the many wonderful evenings that she had enjoyed partying in high society. Her stories of Abigail's life among the great and the good were enchanting, and it was heart-warming to hear of the fun they had all had together.

'Oh my God, did she like to party,' her friend laughed. 'Abigail was one of those girls who never wanted to go home.'

We could organize home help and her friends could arrange a rota to call on her, but Abigail required around-the-clock care. She would need to be transferred to a suitable nursing home – exactly what she had resisted for so long.

It was tragic to see this faded beauty, so vivacious throughout her long and fun-filled life, now lying child-like in a geriatric ward, dependent on people to feed and wash her. Was this why we kept people alive? Is this not exactly what I would hate for myself?

I have to admit I can get frustrated and even angry when I see people like Abigail. Doctors are accused of 'playing God' and yet, if that were the case, what would such a God deem to be kind? It seems cruel to me to keep people alive just because we can. I am not advocating euthanasia, of course, but sometimes it just seems unfair to put old, sick people through even more suffering and indignities.

I asked her friend what she thought and she said, 'The Abigail I knew would have hated this. At least she seems unaware of the world around her, which is a blessing, I suppose.'

I asked why she thought Geoffrey was so against putting a DNR order in place.

'Guilt,' she said. 'They never got along that well, and now he is probably trying to make amends.'

I felt sorry for Geoffrey now too. He was facing the death of his mother with so much unresolved, and yet whatever he might say to her now would fall on deaf ears. He could not fix whatever damage had been done, and now he was facing the rest of his life wondering where their relationship had gone wrong. It was a heavy burden to bear.

Whatever God there might be intervened a few weeks later. We were trying to arrange a nursing home for Abigail, but this can take weeks or months, so she remained on the geriatric ward oblivious to the rotation of fellow patients around her. Her friend visited her one Saturday afternoon and brought her into town.

'She seemed as well as I had seen her in months,' she told me later. 'We had a great day, although I am not sure how much she was able to take in.'

That Saturday night, at about midnight, Abigail stopped breathing. The nurses called the arrest team who arrived en masse and did their best to restore her to life. They were unsuccessful and I only hope Abigail was dead long enough before the team arrived to not care any longer.

CONCLUSION

One of the most brilliant things about neurology and studying the brain and its dysfunction is that you learn at least one new thing about it every day. Every week at our radiology meeting I will, without fail, see something new on a brain scan or hear a suggested diagnosis from a colleague that I either did not think of or had not seen before. Or I might learn a new technique for taking pictures of the brain or a new way of approaching a patient's problem.

The flip side of knowing a little more with each passing year, and meeting thousands of patients, is that you understand just how unclear things relating to the brain can be. Yes, I recognize most patterns of most neurological ailments at this stage, but as soon as I think I have a pattern locked down, I get caught out. And if I'm still seeing the occasional rare case for the first time, and learning something new every day, that is something I did not know the week or the month or the year before. That means the next question you have to ask yourself is, 'Could I have missed something?'

So the older you get the more the false confidence of youth dissipates and you start to realize how much you do not know. That is not to say I do not know what I am doing – I certainly believe I do – but it is truly astonishing, after twenty-five years in the job, to contemplate the breadth and depth of what there is to know, and what is yet to be discovered, about the brain. I fear we will never know all that there is to know about the brain and, in part, that is why studying neurology remains so exciting.

As doctors become more specialized, we know more and more about less and less of the mountains of information we learned years ago in medical school. It is almost impossible to keep up with developments in one's own area, let alone in those of others. So it is understandable that when a doctor sends you to a specialist that their line of thinking – and thus of diagnosis – will lean towards their own area of expertise. In other words, surgeons perform surgery, so that's likely to be what they will have to offer. Analogous to that, my colleagues would be quick to say, is the old joke about neurology . . .

'What do you expect when you go to see a neurologist?'

'Nothing!'

(I hope by now you'll realize that the stereotype is a little unfair.)

I often reflect on what it is we are trying to achieve as doctors. First, we want to save lives that are in immediate danger. When that happens, we are exultant – for a very short while. Then we try to return the sick to health. When that happens we are pleased. But when someone appears to have recovered physically from a neurological condition we are much more limited in our power to return them fully to their pre-patient lives. We can only do so much when someone is ready to return to full health, which can be a long process. That depends on the individual, their friends and families, and on their reactions to the illness. We can assist with physiotherapy and rehabilitation, and psychological support to a degree, but this is hugely limited by clinics so busy that when someone leaves our care we have to focus on the next, and possibly sicker, person. We want to let them go, but sometimes they are fearful and don't want us to. Is that a success? I'm not so sure.

When I sat down to write this book I had not planned to talk about my father or his career. But the more I thought about my life as a doctor, the more intensely I felt his influence, perhaps because I am now of an age to put myself in his shoes. I am certainly able to appreciate how patient and supportive he was when I was setting out as a callow young medical student. I may not have his endless patience, but I learned from him the importance of kindness and courtesy and listening to people, and I hope I bring some of that into my own work. It is something I aspire to do every day.

One thing that has changed for the better since my father's time is the relationship between older and younger doctors. When I regularly catch myself laughing with medical students and younger doctors now, I feel the emotional-intelligence gap has narrowed considerably between my generation and the ones behind me. In my early years as a consultant we would socialize with the younger crowd and it was always great fun. (It happens less now as I get older, simply because

I cannot keep up!) The barriers that I perceived were there between my generation and my father's generation might not have been there at all, but it was certainly not common for myself, or my peers, to chat so candidly or to socialize at all with our seniors when we were in training. Because all that has changed, thankfully, and also because I teach students and young doctors, I think I have a good sense of how life is for the up-and-coming generations of doctors. I am aware of their nervousness, and their bravado, at times. But I love to see the pride in young doctors' faces when they get excited about their work.

I tell students and junior doctors today to try not to be in the same sort of hurry as I was – it is a life-long career with so much to learn along the way. From my class in college, we all appear to be relatively happy to have chosen medicine as a career, which is pretty remarkable considering that most of us started medical school in our late teens. Was it luck or down to perseverance that it worked out for us? Or is it a sense of 'we have come this far and we cannot do anything else'? I am sure that, like myself, former classmates have had periods of self-doubt. It is one of the few remaining 'jobs for life', and if you do not like it, or it does not turn out to suit you, you only find out after six years in college and at least a few years as a junior doctor. In other words, most people do not truly know if they are happy to continue as a doctor until they are at least in their late twenties, by which time a change of career seems terribly daunting.

I recall my father feeling a slight sense of distance from the community and how he talked about the image of doctors when he was coming into the profession – they were seen then as aloof and serious types, a bit unapproachable. I believe that this is much less often the case today, and that the fact we are as subject to the highs and lows of life as the next person is evident to most people.

I wonder what my father would make of how we do medicine now. I certainly think he would have his hands full with increasing bureaucracy and the expectation of constant availability. The opportunity to switch off has practically disappeared in the era of emails and text messages. It is also an ethical minefield. For instance, if someone sends you an email with scan results after hours on a Friday, they feel they have passed on the information and the proverbial ball is now in your court.

What can you do about it on a Friday night? Call a patient with bad news but no solution? Call them, frighten the bejesus out of them, and send them in to sit on a trolley for the weekend 'just in case' something happens before Monday? Or hold the information in among your own anxieties until you can actually do something helpful on Monday morning? Of course, if a scan indicates something critically amiss you are glad to have the information and to act straight away – it's probably something you were chasing urgently anyway. It's the emails or texts in the grey area that eat into your headspace at a time when you should be trying to let go of the stresses of work and renewing your energies. And that is vital for those of us who work with the ill and the dying on a daily basis – not just for our own well-being and the avoidance of burnout, but so we can do our best for our patients.

It is in the nature of many medics to worry that they will get one of the conditions they have studied for years. For many neurologists this is always a deep-seated and heavily denied concern. When you're tired and stressed and your eye muscles flicker (myokymia to the likes of me), you worry you're getting MS. When the muscles of your calf flicker spontaneously, it's motor neuron disease. When you are run down and your hand trembles as you pour your Sunday morning cup of tea, it's inevitable your darker thoughts turn to Parkinson's.

When I tell stories about patients' groundless worries and misguided internet safaris, it is not to criticize them but because I feel their anxiety so acutely. I can only imagine the fear that some people have coming to visit someone like me. I readily admit to a range of phobias of my own, and one that dates back to my teenage years is a trip to the dentist. I have had a kind, calm and competent dentist for the best part of my life. Despite his best efforts, I dread every visit. It's not necessarily the pain, I've decided, but the vulnerability and loss of control that are the root of my fears. When I am stressed I tend to get a pain in one of my back teeth. Convinced I am going to lose a tooth, I arrange to see my poor dentist, who almost invariably reassures me there is nothing to worry about, and the pain magically subsides thereafter. Even neurologists get psychosomatic symptoms.

There is no one-size-fits-all when it comes to a medical condition. Many are reluctant to believe doctors when told that they have the mild end of the disease spectrum. A persistent cough could be due to a bad cold, the flu, pneumonia or lung cancer. How many of us think lung cancer after we google 'persistent cough' and how many of us are reassured that it is, in fact, merely a cold?

Happily, the majority of patients coming to see me for the first time do not have anything serious and are quickly reassured, some more easily than others, but the end result for most is that their mild shaking hands wax and wane at times of stress but do not progress to anything serious. Their stories are no less interesting in terms of the psychology of the mind. They are just as worried as the person who does indeed end up with a serious diagnosis.

One day the sky will fall in on each of us. I urge you to celebrate the fact when today is not that day. While I do not ascribe to 'living every day as if it were your last' – after all, most of us cannot throw in our jobs, spend our savings on a sun-soaked beach and take to the drink – many of the people I meet are spending their one turn on life's merry-go-round obsessing about the potential illness that will stop the ride.

As for those patients for whom the news is not so good, well, the curse of neurodegenerative disorders, particularly MS and Parkinson's, is that neither the doctor nor the patient can be terribly confident in predicting how an individual will get on in the future. You can give statistics, but who knows where a given patient will lie on the statistical curve – the good side or the bad side of the average? Many people find the 'not knowing' tormenting in itself, while others try to get on with their lives with, say, an irritating tremor, not knowing whether it will later incapacitate them or not.

Neurological symptoms are potentially calamitous physically, but also psychologically, and not just to the unwell person, but also to their parents, spouses, children – their entire lives and those of all around them. The immense pleasure at seeing someone who could not walk make a slow but sure recovery is regularly countered by those patients we see who do not recover. Many can no longer hold their children or spouse and they may become dependent on others for the rest of their lives. Making these diagnoses on a daily basis reminds me just how fickle fate can be and how fragile is our humanity. And though I don't always succeed, it prompts me to try to worry less about the ultimately fleeting problems that keep me awake at night. Life really is short and precious.

I find myself thinking almost constantly about the people I see each day. I marvel at how their brain had abruptly, and seemingly without any warning, ceased to work. Or how a person's perfectly ordinary life gradually imploded over the course of many months before they came to see me. I think about our consultation, how it went, and their treatment. I think about my patients' relationships, work and life – and about my own.

Beyond life's leaking pipes and dodgy cars, doctors are forever worried by our choices in others' care, more so than we celebrate the victories. So, no matter how we try to decompress, or switch off, or compartmentalize, we rarely stop thinking about the patients. Ultimately they are why we get up in the morning.

ACKNOWLEDGEMENTS

I have wanted to write about the daily highs and lows of life as a doctor on the frontline of patient care for many years. But I was self-conscious about doing so and it was only with the encouragement of others that I finally got the confidence to go ahead.

Noel Kelly gave me the final push to submit my initial stories for consideration, and he and Niamh Tyndall have been a tremendous support in this endeavour.

Michael McLoughlin, MD at Penguin Random House Ireland, surprised me by suggesting the stories would be worth publishing and editor Nora Mahony was a great help in putting some structure to my otherwise scattered early drafts.

Patricia Deevy at Penguin Ireland has been an incredible support throughout this process and has quietly steered me away from some of my initial thoughts, much to my now relief. I cannot thank her enough for her insights into the world of publishing, a world that was hitherto completely alien to me.

I thought friends might laugh at the thought of me writing a book and I was very relieved when they offered nothing but encouragement, so thanks to all of you – Bart, David BH, David O'D, Catherine, Kieran, Maurice, Gilda, Brian K, David L, Fiona, Eamonn, and friends from Smyth's, among others.

Similarly, I was surprised but delighted that colleagues were so supportive when I mentioned I was writing about our lives as doctors in Ireland. To a man and woman they encouraged me when I was more than a little nervous about things. I admire all the doctors, nurses, receptionists, telephonists, therapists and porters I work with on a daily basis and I hope some of them might see aspects of themselves in this book – the highs as well as the lows – and know how much I appreciate their commitment to our patients. Thanks especially to Joe and Jackie and, of course, to Paula C who helps keep me sane.

ACKNOWLEDGEMENTS

Heartfelt thanks to Bellini who is the real writer and yet did nothing but encourage me when the book became a reality. I will forever cherish the many great times we have shared together.

I would especially like to thank my mother and my elder sister Judith who have been a great support throughout all of our lives and have helped us as a family remain as close as we are.

I meet my brothers Ryan and Garrett and sister Rachel on a weekly basis to chat about life, the world and the universe. It was at one of those meetings that the suggestion I write was first made and it was only with their support that I did not feel as foolish or narcissistic about writing a book as I might otherwise have done. I look forward to our few quiet beers every week and I cannot thank them enough for all they do for me.